TODDLER DISCIPLINE FOR EVERY STAGE

Written By

Jennifer Siegel

Table of Contents

INTRODUCTION

Thank you for purchasing this book!

<u>Break Up The Action Or Cool Down</u>

The age of 24 months (2 years old), communication, physical, and socialization skills of children are blossoming. This "terrible two" stage is not a joke. It is the age of tantrums or emotional thunderstorms, which is a cue to be more consistent with the limits and rules you set to prevent him from adopting a harmful habit.

Time-out is an effective way to calm down the child's overwhelming emotions and break the cycle of malicious behavior. It is a useful calming tool when alternatives, reasoning, and calmness does not work. It provides a chance for both of you to cool down, sending a clear message to the child that adverse action is not the right way to get your attention.

However, do not forget that time outs should not last more than two minutes or until your toddler calms down. It is essential to avoid making him feel rejected, abandoned, confused, and frightened, which will cause more occurrences of power struggles. Always keep in mind the rule of thumb when employing the time-out- 1 minute per year of his age. When the time is up, tell him to come back to his usual play are and reconnect with him.

You can also try the alternative of time-out, which is the time-in. It is a positive form of relaxation that you can use during the epic meltdown moments. The idea is to invite the child to sit somewhere with you near him, allowing him to cool down and express his feelings. The parent is encouraged to show empathy without saying something- just building a slow connection until the showdown is over. Once he is calm, it's time to connect and discuss what happened, allowing him to spill out his emotions and help him find a solution to ensure that it will not happen again.

Advantages of time-in strategy:

- It keeps the connection before the presentation of correction.

- It makes the child feel that his need is being considered.

- It provides time for the child to process his emotions.

- It makes him feel secure, understood, and not alone during the crucial moments.

- It prevents a power struggle that usually comes with a time-out.

Enjoy your reading!

Mind Development

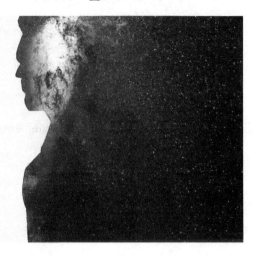

Everything we learn reaches the brain through our senses. But the mind has built-in barriers to the entry of sensory information. It is a beautiful organ, but unable to process the billions of bits of information that bombard it every second. To handle the dam, it is equipped with filters to protect against input overload and focuses on the most critical data for survival. The way your child's brain responds to sensitive environmental information determines what information gets your attention. Only selected data passes through your lower brain filter (called the reticular activation system or RAS) to enter your thinking brain. The RAS is especially sensitive to newspapers, surprises, color, and unexpected/curious events when choosing a sensory input to allow for thinking.

Once the information passes through the first filter, there is a second filter in the part of the brain called the tonsil. The amygdala is part of the network of the limbic system that processes emotions. The way your child stores sensory information passing through the tonsil filter is vastly inflated by his emotional state when he receives the information. When stress is high, the tonsil redirects the data to an automatic reflex system, dominated by non-reflex reactions, such as theft. When the amygdala is in a safe condition, and emotions are positive, information is transferred to the brain, creating networks of memory and reflection. There is something that helps sensory input pass through these two filters: a chemical neurotransmitter named dopamine. When learning is connected with pleasure, dopamine is released. This boost increases concentration, helping the brain to stay awake. As a parent, understanding how information enters the brain to become knowledge and long-term memory is an excellent tool for enriching your child's mind. Using brain-tailored strategies allows your child to respond to the most useful sensory information in their environment and transform that information into stored knowledge.

RAD Learning

There are two essential brain processes and three major brain systems that are key to developing a better brain. The methods are structuring and neuroplasticity. Three plans are what I call RAD, which is the abbreviation for:

R: reticular activation system (RAS)

A: Affective filter in the amygdala

D: Dopamine

The Science Behind Better Learning

Reticular Activation System (RAS) - The brain control panel of the RAS is a switching system that activates the attention located in the lower brain (brain). It's SAR selectively alerts the brain to changes in its environment that affect their survival: sounds, images, and smells that may indicate danger or indicate opportunities to find food, a partner, or refuge.

In humans, RAS has evolved to become more sensitive to basic needs than to survival in nature, but it remains a filter that is more attentive to changes in our environment. RAS is the key to activating the level of reaction and alertness in the brain. The RAS's response to the sensory information it receives dictates the speed, content, and kind of information available to the "superior" mind. Although millions of bits of sensory data blast RAS every second of waiting, this filter limits access to about two thousand bits per second.

In successful learning, children are encouraged to draw attention to important information by attracting the attention of their RAS. Listening to lectures and exercises and worksheets are not new or exciting experiences, so they do not contain enough sensory stimulation to feed information through RAS filters in the brain.

<u>Dopamine</u>

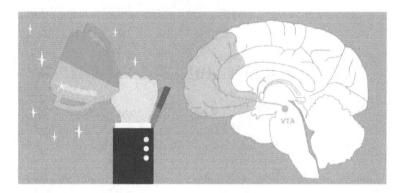

Dopamine is one of the brain's most significant neurotransmitters. (A portion of different neurotransmitters in the brain incorporate serotonin, tryptophan, acetylcholine, and norepinephrine.) These neurotransmitters are synthetic brain substances that convey information over the spaces (neurotransmitters) that structure when one nerve finishing interfaces with another. During the last trimester of fetal advancement, the brain makes thirty thousand neural connections for each second for each square centimeter of the cortical surface.

The brain discharges dopamine when an encounter is pleasurable. As a pleasure-chasing organ, the brain likewise releases dopamine in desire for fulfilling, enjoyable encounters. This has a few preferences.

Dopamine discharges increments of mindful focus and memory arrangement. At the point when dopamine is released during pleasant learning exercises, it expands children's abilities to control consideration and store long term recollections.

Learning activities that can initiate the arrival of dopamine and make pleasurable states in the brain incorporate physical development, individual interest associations, social contacts, music, curiosity, feeling of accomplishment, characteristic prize, decisions, play, and funniness. The dopamine discharged during these exercises is then accessible to build consideration and focus.

Inner inspiration is significant in objective setting and driving forward with schoolwork, examining, and focus in class. Significantly when the objectives are identified with individual interest, children will expand on their qualities and appreciate the dopamine-pleasure reaction from their objective coordinated accomplishments. A considerable lot of the techniques in this book are associated with building dopamine-pleasure brain reactions.

Amygdala

The sensory information that children get—the things they see, hear, feel, smell, or touch—invigorates the admission focuses of their brains past the RAS. The zones most dynamic when new information first enters the mind are the sensory cortex territories in every flap of the mind. This information is recognized and grouped by coordinating it with recently put-away comparable data. Seeing a lemon, for instance, interfaces with the visual cortex in the occipital flaps. The feel of the lemon is perceived by the somatosensory (touch) that focuses on the parietal projections.

This sensory data should then go through the brain's intense center, the limbic system, particularly the amygdala and hippocampus, where enthusiastic criticalness is linked to information (acrid taste is yummy in lemon sherbet however yucky in unsweetened lemon juice). On accepting sensory data, these exciting filters assess their pleasure esteem. That choice decides whether the information is given further access to the higher brain, and assuming this is, that's where the data will go. At the point when the brain sees danger or the child feels focused on, these brain channel focuses go into survival mode and redirect the sensory data from the thinking mind and into the programmed focuses (battle/flight). Since there are usually no tigers in our homes, children genuinely needn't bother with a similar danger channel reaction their ancient ancestors did. However, those filters still exist in human brains and can be initiated by the sort of stresses children have with specific study halls.

Tormenting, consideration challenges, confusion, or boredom may trigger these filters, obstructing the ingestion of sensory information identified with learning. The battle/flight reaction is locked because the boosts are seen as negative encounters, and knowledge gets troublesome. If your child is disappointed, exhausted, or confused because she realizes how to duplicate parts, yet is doing one more worksheet increasing portions, or if she's confused by the troublesome jargon words in the story the class is perusing, her amygdala reacts to those worries by taking up a significant part of the brain's accessible supplements and oxygen. The mind, at that point, goes into survival mode.

16

The high movement in the amygdala squares the area of information to the thinking brain and memory. This is the reason learning methodologies that lessen children's nervousness are significant: They bring down the full of a feeling (passionate) channel in the amygdala and enable information to arrive at the thinking focuses. At the point when your child is focused on, the amygdala guides knowledge to the responsive, no thinking brain. At the point when your child is loose, agreeable, and interested, the amygdala directs the information to the intelligent, thinking mind. At the point when you comprehend the elements of these filters, you can likewise utilize them in positive manners. If learning encounters are related to pleasure, associated with themes of interest, or identified with fulfilling objective accomplishment and other positive encounters, sensory data will be viewed as an essential and allowed area into the higher, thinking brain. With well-arranged learning exercises that support consideration and interest without delivering dissatisfaction, confusion, or boredom, these filters can be enrolled to enable the mind to concentrate on the sensory information of the learning movement. Alongside the amygdala in the limbic system is the hippocampus.

It is in this solidification focus that new sensory information is linked to past details and to recollections of past encounters recovered from memory stockpiling. Positron outflow tomography (PET) filters show that when children are given new information, their brains actuate their put-away memory banks. Their minds look for connections or associations between the further information and put-away recollections of past knowledge or experience. At the point when new information is combined with an earlier report, the recently coded social memory is currently prepared for handling the frontal projections and long haul memory stockpiling.

The Brain

It has higher thinking networks that process new information through what is called official capacities, including judgment, investigation, organizing, and essential leadership. It is in the official capacity networks that further information is mentally controlled to become a memory. At the point when your child's prefrontal cortex effectively forms new communication with mental manipulation, for example, critical thinking, arranging, or predicting, his official capacities take responsibility for further details, and it is changed from short-term into long-term memory.

At the point when your child's brain transforms sensory contribution to memory, she learns. The development of new recollections enables her mind to remember my experience and predict the result of her conduct. Memory is a survival necessity for creatures that must learn, store, and recall how they ought to respond to physical needs and changes in their conditions. They reactivate stored recollections to reflect and predict. Where did they go to find nourishment? What were spots hazardous due to predators? Where was the protected cavern that gives a safe house?

Each time your child remembers something, he is likewise reactivating a neural system that his brain recently made. At the point when he adds new recollections identified with information as of now in brain stockpiling, the neural circuit for that example or class of information develops more significant as more associations structures between nerve cells. The more data stored in the brain's networks, the more effectively we respond to our surroundings. The more we learn, the more data stored in our neural networks, the more probable our brains are to identify with new information—henceforth, learning advances learning.

Communication

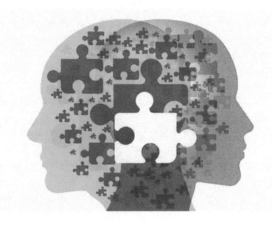

Communication with your child represents an open door. The child will often initiate a conversation (sometimes it can be an open invitation for help), but the question is whether you will recognize this call for help, hear it, and answer it with an adequate response. If you invest in communicating with your child, this communication becomes the foundation for building a lasting relationship.

Some Of The Fundamental Laws Of Good Communication With Your Child Are:

Consider their age. You can already explain the "great" secrets of life to your three-year-old child. It is surprising, but your toddler can understand how children are born, whether there is a God, what happens when someone dies, and similar things. Still, when you are talking to a child, the principle is always the same: tell the truth using words the child is already familiar with.

Communication is a two-way street when you share your everyday experiences with a child rather than expecting them to talk to you. If you get a detailed answer to how your toddler spent the day, the child deserves to receive a detailed response to his question.

Share your personal opinions. You don't have to always keep things in confidence just because of the different levels of a child's thinking. On the contrary, it is your duty still to state your opinion, that is, what you believe to be right, but in a manner that does not hurt your child, does not diminish him or her, or underestimate him. Just talk.

Always show your child enough patience and time to talk. If your toddler grows up with the conviction that he still has contacts with his parents - he will feel safer and happier. Try setting priorities. If your toddler wants to talk to you while doing some housework, let your child do so.

Communication is learned. Occasional quarrels, conflicts, and misunderstandings are ordinary and typical occurrences in touch. But never give up.

Speech is given to us, but the conversation is learned. We all can hear, but to understand, we have to put effort, time, and love into learning to listen.

How To Control The Child's Aggression

From time to time, your child gets bruises and scratches from taking a fall and playing games with their friends. Children have always played "mother and daughter" and "catch." It might seem like you could say to your child: "Give the doll to Katie; you're a girl!" But even if your child does it, you may not know what feelings are at work inside her: maybe she will get the impression that it's not so good to be good.

If you see or suspect how difficult it is for a two-year-old child to part with their favorite toy for the sake of good manners, it is better not to push the child and not to bring on hysterics.

When your toddler becomes a little older and has more experience in communicating, it will be calmer for him or her to focus in similar situations, and as far as possible – to try to predict them.

Often, parents are afraid of another type of situation, in which their child might be aggressive, taking a toy from another child. Almost all kids struggle if they are somewhat dissatisfied and misbehave if they are tired. Sometimes the aggressiveness of the child takes the form of your toddler biting other children.

This is the same situation.

As long as a quarrel doesn't lead to outright aggression on the part of one or more children, parents should not interfere. If there is a need to intervene, do not try to find the culprit: for one of the children, your decision will still be unfair.

It is better to separate the fighters and divert their attention to other activities. If you see that one of the children is continually tormenting your child, look for another circle of friends, at least for some time, where the relationship between children will be somewhat different.

Perhaps your toddler is too small to respect other children. This respect needs to be learned gradually. Take the child aside and, at the same time, explain that the other child is hurt and that your child needs to apologize to him or her. If there is an opportunity, let your bully play with older children- in that type of situation, it will be harder for them to prove their strength. Note: the older the child, the more selective your toddler will be in demonstrating his aggressiveness towards other people. Children are most likely aware of when they can get away with it and when they cannot.

In any case, children should be taught systematically to share toys.

If your child reveals an aggressiveness that frightens you, you have to think: perhaps, its origins lie in the relationships that have developed in your family. Don't forget that you are an example to your child. And yet, the skills of exhibiting a right attitude towards each other are better instilled when the child is in good humor.

Outpouring Of Feelings

Teach your toddler to be concerned about everyone around them. Let them help you during cooking: put the dishes on the table with you, put out bread and fruit. And it would help if you accompanied their actions with encouraging words. Of course, it will take more time to do the work than if the child wasn't "disturbing you," but you have learned that feeding a child is not all there is to raising him or her. Remember this.

You might put a doll or a toy animal down to sleep, gently stroking them "before bed," saying that they've been good and obedient. Ask your toddler to show how he or she loves the doll or toy animal.

Show your toddler how to take care of flowers, paying attention to the fact that they have beautiful small and delicate leaves and flowers.

When you go for a walk, take food for birds or squirrels in the park, feed them together, and praise the toddler for it.

If the child is sad or over-excited, he won't do what you ask of him (maybe he will break a leaf or throw a doll on the floor or won't want to feed the animals).

This temporary act of aggression does not indicate lousy character traits at all.

A sense of parental love and tenderness allows a child to feel good and desired and gives him or her confidence in life.

What Is Right And What Is Wrong

While a baby is small, the parents' main prohibitions are related to the concern for their safety. When forbidding something and saying the word "No," do not forget to explain why and tell the child how to do what he needs to do. Also, parents should know that praise is much more instructive than prohibiting things.

As often as possible, show approval for the good things your toddler does, especially those that were hard for them. Do not merely give them prohibitions. According to psychologists, a verbal ban is not meant for a child up to five years old.

The best solution to any problem is its joint discussion. If possible, examine the forbidden object that interests the baby together. Remembering the child's age, try to find an explanation to show him what the danger is.

Suppose you need to take something away from your toddler and not let them use it, offer something to replace it, but always with something new or exciting. In most cases, conflict can be avoided.

It is advisable for adults involved in the upbringing of a child to discuss the limits allowed so that, as the toddler grows, he or she will not be confused: if dad considers this acceptable, why does grandma forbid it?

26

But do not do this in the presence of the toddler. And even when being guided by safety considerations, allow several things to the child in a row. This can destroy the child's desire for initiative or cause them excessive nervousness.

A child's desire to touch something with his hands or taste it isn't always due to mischief (as sometimes it seems to parents). This is the typical desire that a child has to know the world around him and gain their own experience.

Try not to say to a child: "You are bad!" Instead, say: "You did a bad thing!" Even if your toddler does not understand everything, your attitude towards him and your tone of voice can clarify the meaning of what is happening.

Analyze the reasons for the conflicts that arise: is it possible that you are annoyed by seeing in your child a character trait that you have been trying to get rid of yourself for a long time?

When children are happy with everything, they usually behave well, but sometimes they unconsciously want to push the limits. At this time, it seems to parents that the child is testing their patience.

Often, bad behavior is a way to attract attention. The child may try to establish himself as being in opposition to the adults he continually communicates. If you see the child is very enthusiastic in an activity, try not to interrupt it, even if it's time to eat or sleep.

Help them finish their "business," and then offer whatever is needed. The child will get used to spending what he is doing.

The most sensible way to resist hysterics and fits is to ignore them if they become habitual. Stay calm and kind with your child, but firmly insist on your authority, and in the end, your toddler will understand that lying on the floor in hysterics is not the best way to win an argument.

Sometimes a child needs some help to stop the hysteria.

Each family has its ways of settling disobedience, based on their experience of communicating with the child.

Try to be guided by these principles:

A child is a full member of the family (but not the center of it).

The child has the right to his own opinion (even if your toddler does not speak yet) - and this should be taken into account.

Just like an adult, the child has the right to a bad mood: from time to time, they may be angry, maybe dissatisfied, or may cry. It is not always because of external circumstances.

Tantrum

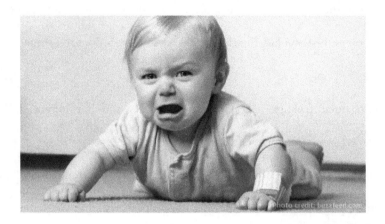

Tantrums are a relatively natural aspect of a child's life from around one year to 5 years of age. Let's hope they start a little later than one year and finish sooner, but everything in this range is relatively standard. Your kid discovers that events don't necessarily go their way. And as guardians, we need to help them know how to cope with these feelings and make amends.

It may not be comforting for a parent. It's hard to know when your child is calling for your support. We feel stressed by the situation and need help to settle down. Now isn't the time to take things seriously.

When to prevent tantrums: it can be essential to stop tantrums until the child loses power. Here are few suggestions to fend off tantrums as you see your child's first losing control symptoms.

How To Avoid Tantrums

1. Be careful – carry a little bag with a few easy games and some fun treats if you want your kid to wait unwearyingly for a doctor's surgery or a coffee shop.

2. Mark their feelings—"Boy, you wish you could live longer"—"You needed some orange juice right now! "

3. Redirect them—"I can't let you strike your dad, but you can strike the drum/pillow."

4. Get down to their level, "You sound irritated. Would you give me that? "

5. When they're hurting, ask them when they'd like any support – give them as much encouragement as they want, and then stand back.

6. Give them an option – "Would you prefer to put your shoes or scarf on first? "

7. Establish routines—"And we'll go to the bathroom after lunch, read a novel, and have some rest."

8. Let them display their frustration in a fun way, "Tell me how mad you are. Here's a sheet of paper and a pencil. Yeah. Wow. They're broad circles. You're too nuts! "

<u>Triggers</u>

Problems will always intensify to a full-blown tantrum. Often, it's because of your child's frustration, anger, or rage; they often want to be in control; their contact can be limited; or because they're sleepy, starving, or over-stimulated. They will throw themselves on the floor, drive us aside, reach us/sister/other kids, or even smash something.

This might be useful to remember items that induce tantrums in your child: over-scheduling could be standard; a new baby; going home; even other children can activate this.

Often, the tantrum is triggered by us, when we're offering the news that it's time to quit the playground, or that we're preparing any food they don't want for dinner, or whether we'd like them to get ready and leave the house.

It's all right for your kid to hold a tantrum. It would be best if you accepted their frustration with what's going on. Please don't make them do anything they don't want. If we sit back down and give way to them, you'll note that they will cry much more often every time.

It's hard to be a parent and remain stable. Yet the diligent work is going to pay off in the long term. They'll know that when you say no, you mean no, and when you say yes, you mean no, too:).

I like the suggestion from "Good Discipline: The Baby Years": "If you say it, you believe it; and if you think it, carry up with caring and strict practice" Practice could be, for example, leaving the park with an unhappy child, knowing that they wish they could linger longer.

Alternatives to time out – how to make your child settle down While your child has a tantrum, several psychologists suggest you take time out. I consider this frustrating because your child is calling for assistance to settle down, so withdrawing your support at this moment isn't a wise approach.

If we discipline our children, they sometimes get upset at us rather than being sad about what they have done. Or they'll try to find out a way to get away with it next time without getting identified.

Then, I search for opportunities to help my kid settle down. I don't assume that their action is all right. Perhaps it's not possible to tell them anything while they're in the midst of the tantrum. They're not around to understand you. They've lost track of things.

Helping Them Calm Down

Some kids are going to need cuddling during a tantrum. You should massage their heads, cuddle them, and sing to them while they go through all kinds of feelings, from rage, deep disappointment, sorrow, and even to remorse. I used to carry my son for

40 minutes because he declined to get ready. So I was watching him go through all these feelings.

Some kids are going to drive you backward and don't want to be treated. In this situation, I make sure they're healthy, so they can't harm themselves or others. Then I stay alongside then start to offer my support, "I'm here if you need any help to settle down. Or maybe we'll have a cuddle when you're ready. "I want to cuddle the tantrum. "It was brutal. And now you've cooled down. Will you like to get a hug? "If they throw toys at their siblings or attempt to reach me, I'll withdraw from them so that everyone is healthy. "I can't let you get me right now. My health is essential to me. Do you like to touch some pillows instead? "When they're going to harm the kid, you should physically put yourself in them and protect the child while you help them settle down.

Older kid: You should set up a "calm spot" for kids over three years of age that they can use while they're upset. It might be a tent with a few pillows and their favorite things. This might be a corner with several ships. You may ask them if they want to go to their quiet spot.

This is separate from the moment the child is in control; they will come forward as they are relaxed. If they're always coming back still angry, I'd politely remind them that they look like they need to cool down to go back when they're able.

Making Amends

One might believe that if I comfort my kid as they settle down, I'm convincing them that their action is ok, so I allow them to get upset. When they're mad, my job is to help them settle down.

When they're calm, I then help them make changes. When they wanted to draw on the ground, I ask them to help me pick up. When they destroyed the toy of their dad, they could help repair it. I begged the kids to help clean their sheets after using the marker pens in their room and creating a mess.

They learn to accept accountability in this manner when things go wrong.

So when it's over, it's over: the positive part for small children is that they will switch quickly from intense frustration or disappointment back to their happier self. We ought to pass forward, though, and not allow something to disrupt the entire day by going back to or following up with it.

When The Changes Have Been Made, It's Safe For Us To Carry On:

Aren't We All Meant To Forgive Their Tantrum?

When they have tantrums, I don't like to neglect a child. They don't let me near them, but I keep providing help and making them realize that I'm available anytime they need me. If you're outraged and your friend had left the room to get over it, you'd still consider them abandoned. We tell our children whether they're friendly or wrong, we're going to be there for them.

What Am I Going To Say While We're Out In Public While They Have A Tantrum?

Essentially, there are two options:

1. Go home – if you find it challenging to convince people to see you, it's better to go. It may involve leaving a massive shopping cart and pursuing the suggestions above while you're done.

2. Stay to help them – my favorite choice is to stick in and do as you should do even if you're out of the building. So then provide as much support as you can to help your child settle down. People watching are most inclined to talk of what a wonderful, caring parent you are, rather than what an awful noise your kid is making.

I Consider It Hard To Hold Myself Cool. How Should I Deal With It?

When you've been upset by your kids, it's tough to help them settle down.

- When your companion is eligible, it might be better to get them to move in instead.
- You may want to make sure the children are healthy and run to the toilet to catch your breath.

- Use a quote that you should use, "I breathe softly, I breathe out my frustration."

- Try not to take it personally. You may want to imagine throwing on a bullet-resistant suit that can withstand everything (including words) that your child throws at you.

Conflict Resolution From Tantrums To Tranquility

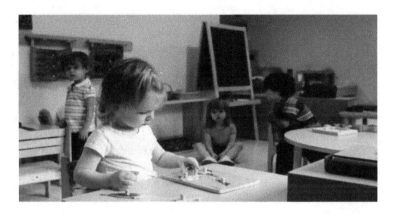

Imagine having a wonderful day with your child. You go to the zoo, you have a nice lunch, and you joke and play together all day. On the way home, you stop at the store, and your child asks for a candy bar. After all the sweets they had at the zoo, you decide it is in their best interest to say "no simply." Cue meltdown.

The entirety of the day seems like it was almost wasted by your child's chosen way to react to this simple refusal of a candy bar. What is it that was holding the two of you from having the perfect day? The answer lies within the communication you have—all determined by the boundaries that have been set lastly.

When you can start to communicate clearly with your child, it becomes easier to live a more tranquil life. You do not just set boundaries for right now; you do so that you and your child can hope for a happier and healthier life as time goes on.

Like other skills that need to be learned, excellent communication with your child is a skill that has to be taken into deliberation, and over time, you get better. You already know that conversation with your children requires being a good listener and talking in some ways that encourage excellent listening skills from your child. For a mother to be aware of the best ways to communicate clearly with their child, they are obligated to understand some basics of communication and what communication with your child is all about.

When it comes to collaborating with your child, it involves inviting them to talk to you to express what they are feeling, the ability to listen, and give a response in a sensitive way - positive and negative. You also have to ensure you are paying attention to gestures and tone, including words, to be able to understand better what is being said by them.

Undoubtedly, if you will want an enhanced and improved bond between you and your child, you have to stimulate excellent boundary-setting abilities. With that in mind, I've outlined practical ways you can set boundaries with your child. The three necessary steps include creating a way to talk to each other, listen to what they have to say, and teach them to be good listeners as well.

Setting Boundaries

Setting clear boundaries is crucial for your child. Ensure that you have chosen a specific period that you and your child can communicate and set boundaries with each other. Do not just wait until you are already in the middle of a tantrum. Is your hectic schedule the hindrance to having excellent communication with your child? You are not alone, but it will interest you to know that many have solved that issue by merely utilizing family meals as a way to foster listening and talking.

During that process, what most folks do is talk about things that have happened that day. The more you talk about trivial things, the more you are opening ways for more critical tasks. Also, be open about all sorts of feelings they could have - anxiety, joy, frustration, and fears.

Be familiar with your child's gestures. Practice paying attention to non-audible signals. Is he too quiet? Then ask him what happened and why he's silent. Always strive hard to work together to combat problems. And lastly, emphasize the need, to be honest. Always be keen about speaking the truth, and each time he or she does, commend that genuinely and do not pretend.

Even though they will not seem to make sense most of the time, we must work to listen to our children and what they have to say. Now that you've created time and you've peered into what should be done, it is time to learn how to listen to them when they express themselves. You would not want your child to feel like you are not listening. Therefore, build on what your toddler is trying to say and reveal your interest. You could say: "go on" or say something along the lines of, "tell me more about it." You could even show amazement by saying: "really?"

Also, while your child talks, make it your goal to be a good reader of facial expressions and body language. Try and see what is behind those words that are being spoken. Try and repeat what is being communicated by your child and maintain eye contact. Additionally, be careful not to cut in while he or she says or makes the mistake of putting words into their mouth.

In some situations, you might not need to solve it, just simply listen. And lastly, always push your child to talk to you. If they believe that they have your attention, then they will continue to use that time. This will keep them more satisfied later, when they might feel needy or clingy, and you are not available to give them full attention.

Lastly, you will need to teach your child how they can listen the most efficiently. If you are not actively teaching them that they need to hear you out, then they will start only to be concerned with their thoughts and feelings.

One of the subtle ways to ensure that he is a good listener is by teaching him by your examples. Do not jump into his words; allow him to finish his talks first before you respond. Use language and a speaking pattern that will enhance good comprehension of your comments. Most times, if he does not understand you, paying attention becomes a plea. Ensure that instructions and requests are revealed. Use simple words; time for teaching is quite different from time to learn grammar. Do not blame or overly criticize. When you show judgment, your child will only become more fearful of opening up to you.

There shouldn't be whatsoever holding you back from showing love towards your child by setting clear and explicit limits. The humble fact is that you have to keep remembering that your toddler wants guidelines. It is just part of their learning process. But how would you do it without intruding into their safety and getting them scared? These are things and ways to uphold.

You are required to teach your kids that you are trustworthy. Always back up your words with actions. Your limit and boundaries will become firm. Avoiding having too many, or at least introducing, too many rules at once. Most times, a few limitations and restrictions at a time frame is better than a long list of limits.

Make the boundaries you set clear and understandable, and do not confuse them with language or grammar. Repeat with them so that you can see if they grasp what it means to go to bed at 8, or sweep after they play with crafts, or not try and ride the dog like it is a horse. Do not use words that could be misunderstood. It is never a way to instill a positive environment. To ensure if what you've said is clearly understood, ask them to repeat what they've heard.

One of the most critical boundaries setting rules is to let your child in on the process. You are not a dictatorship, your household is not one under communism, and you shouldn't even look at your family as a democracy. The way that you lead is through positive relationships, not governmental institutions. Give them a chance to have input on the rules and boundaries that you both will be following.

Take your child through the boundary setting stage. Before you start, assemble everyone, get everyone in the boundary setting, ask for their opinions, readjust them, and let them conclude their readjusted statement. Then from there, you can make it a limit. That way, they see it as being the one that sets the standard for what is right, and they will be inclined to harness more. Regardless, do not throw off your duty as the final judge. But let everyone have a part to play.

Consistency

If you want the boundaries you worked so hard to put in place to stick, then you need to ensure that you are reliable with this. Your child will learn on their own that it is OK and even necessary to break the rules every once in a while. It is not about showing them fluidity in what they choose to do. Instead, you are teaching them that they need to stick to their word. You are showing morality, virtue, and this is what can carry your child long distances when they might be struggling to understand certain parts of the world.

Always do what is right, and if you want to be inconsistent for whatever reason, let them know that it is a treat. For example, you might let them stay up later to watch a movie night when it is the weekend, and a friend is over. You might tell them it is OK to have an extra cupcake on their birthdays. Just make sure that any inconsistency is justified and easily explainable and clear to the child.

Everyday Life And Practical Strategies

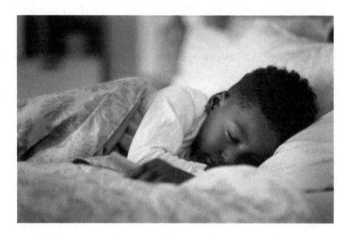

As a toddler is learning, you need to introduce behaviors that he recognizes as part of the going to bed process and a winding down of another day. Your toddler's body clock is not yet set, and all of the steps I have outlined will help you help your toddler establish those links. You can say that "Mr. Clock" says it's time to put the toys away, for example, so that the child does not feel that it's the parent's fault that play has come to an end for the day. Here is the ideal schedule for putting toddlers to bed in perfect circumstances. Bear in mind that you will have to make adjustments when you are traveling when the child is not in his own home and at times of illness, but apart from that, the routine should become something the child becomes familiar with.

Toys Get Put Away

This is a good habit. It clears up the play area and leaves the house tidy. This may be on the ground floor in some homes, and it's important what the place looks like. Invest in a giant toy box instead of expecting a child to sort through things and put them into individual cupboards as that may be a little difficult for the child to grasp. If you have drawing tools, these can all be placed into a plastic box so that they don't stain other things, but at the end of the day, all of the playthings are to be put into the box. Mom can help with the clearing up because toddlers love to mimic adults and will be happier to join in rather than be expected to do all of their work.

Bath And Pajamas

This gets the child into the routine that he needs to be clean and relaxed at the end of the day. If you want to encourage your little ones to enjoy this time, invest in some floating toys and even bubble baths suitable for their delicate skin. This is a time when the child is preparing for what he knows lies ahead, and parents should supervise the bathing process and wash the child's hair. It can be a fun time but don't make it too rowdy as you are also getting ready to wind down for the day.

Supper

It is known that kids who have supper sleep better relating to this. You will see the kind of supper that is usual at this time of night. It is a light something to stop hunger pangs and a drink but not too large. This is enough food for the night and will prevent the child from complaining about being hungry five minutes after being tucked in for the night. Supper should be a time spent sat down eating, rather than being active. If parents can sit down with the kids, this gives them the impression that they are not alone. After supper, make sure that one of you goes upstairs and draws the curtains to the nursery to correct the bedroom ambiance for sleeping. Check the bed and go back down to the children to encourage them to go to the bathroom, clean their teeth, and have one last try to go to the toilet.

Tooth Brushing And Toilet

It's an excellent idea to make sure that your little one has a clean diaper for the night, and this is the ideal time for that. Make sure that your toddler is encouraged to clean his teeth properly and to ready himself for bed. You may find that the child likes a little bit of independence, so I encourage parents to have a stool that the child can stand on. The more grown-up a child feels at this age, the more the child feels in control of learning things like potty training and hygiene, so encourage your child to enjoy this part of the evening.

Choosing Your Reading Material Together

You want to avoid any hurry at this stage. Take your time with your child and choose suitable reading material before placing the child into bed and tucking him. The story should never be something that will wake him/her up but should be read in a low voice, so that the child can hear, but also so that he relaxes while the words are read to him. He may enjoy looking at the pictures, but at bedtime, make this kind of interaction minimal because you don't want to wake him up. You can promise him that you can look through the book tomorrow at playtime, but make sure that you keep the promise as he/she will remember that you made it.

Getting The Room Ready For The Night

The room light should already be subdued, so when the reading is finished, tuck teddy into bed with your little one and ask him/her to look after teddy because teddy needs lots of love. Never skimp on a cuddle before you place the child into bed because, after the reading, all that is left is a little bit of affection and a kiss goodnight. The child knows that you will leave the room, which may prove to be a difficult time with boys. If it is, an extra cuddle won't go amiss, but the child does have to understand that bedtime is bedtime, and there is no negotiation.

Dealing With Crying

It is quite familiar for a child to whimper before they go off to sleep. They are tired, probably a little cranky, and now you are leaving them on their own in their bedroom, which makes their little hearts a bit anxious. However, although you may be monitoring the sounds, be aware that this may die down very quickly if the child is left to it. Some systems have been devised whereby you are told by experts to ignore crying. However, if the crying gets too forceful, the child can get extremely distressed, and I would never recommend that to anyone. Go in and cuddle the child if you have to calm him, but remember that placing the child in his bed for sleep is very important. Any other reaction will encourage the child to keep on trying to win your favor when it comes to being moved into the grown-up's bed.

It would help if you remembered that psychological damage can come from fear and that this battle is about fear, not about wits. If your child is a little uncomfortable with the level of light, perhaps you can adjust the light a little so that he feels more comfortable. Sit on the chair beside the bed. Sing a lullaby if you want to, and you will notice that the child will gradually go to sleep. It may take a little bit of training, but the idea is that you slowly move away from the bed's side. You are still there to reassure, but the distance between you should become more so that you can leave the room and carry on with your evening without too much problem.

Safety Considerations In The Bed Area

Ensure that the bed is not crowded in with toys and that there is nothing that can harm the child within the size of the bed. This should be a cozy place where the child can relax without turning over and hurting himself on sharp toys. You will know from the level of dribbles whether the child is teething, which may give you a clue about the child's discomfort. If you pop in before you go to bed and notice that the pillowcase is particularly wet, you can change it so that the wetness does not disturb your little one while he sleeps.

The reason that you leave changing the diapers until the last moment is so that the child has a chance to get through the night without the diaper becoming uncomfortable or wet or soiled. This helps the child to get off to sleep without the diversion of bodily needs. Most toddlers will respond well to a dry bed and are less likely to be woken by discomfort if the ground is dry, and the diaper is clean.

Catering For The Bodily Needs Of A Toddler

On average, a toddler needs a total of 11 to 12 hours of sleep in 24 hours. Keep a diary note of the times that the child slept in the day, and you will get a much better idea of how to adjust the daytime schedule to encourage more tiredness at night. This will change as the child grows, but for the time being, it's essential that you respect that need and that during the hours of being awake, the child eats food that is nutritious and gets plenty of outdoor exercises. This helps the child to get the healthiest nutrition and fresh air, and all of this contributes to how well the toddler sleeps. A happy child with a well-balanced life will be easier to train than one who is not given sufficient exercise and has excess energy to burn when it comes to bedtime. That extra energy could be the reason for lack of sleep, so adjust the daytime schedule accordingly.

Remember, there is no bargaining when it comes to bedtime. Many parents do barter with their children by saying, "Okay, one more story" or "Okay, you can come downstairs for another half hour," or by letting the child dictate the bedtime rules. It has been proven repeatedly that this isn't the end of the problem but is the beginning. A child who knows that a parent will bargain will be even more angry and upset when the parent decides that bargaining is impossible on certain nights of the week. Thus, you need to instill that just as a child eats his breakfast, he also needs to learn that specific actions are not negotiable. The ideal steps are ones that will get you off to a good start. Involve the toddler in every step, including putting the toys away, sitting very still and quietly for his/her supper, going through the hygiene things like cleaning the teeth, and going to the toilet. The child will have a better understanding of what is to be expected at bedtime.

The things that will sidetrack you are:

- Illness and how to deal with it

- Crying that seems irrational

- Signs that something is wrong and getting to the bottom of it

The child showed • Insecurity in the way he/she acts out

Most of these are common sense things to deal with. For example, if you suspect illness, then a visit to the doctor can reassure you. Crying that seems irrational can be dealt with by sitting by the child's bed and trying to work out what is upsetting the child, without taking the child out of the bedroom environment. Sometimes, the child needs to settle down with the teddy and reassure that mom or dad is there listening to them. You can also go through the different room areas to reassure the child that there is nothing to be afraid of.

Biting, Hitting, And Kicking. What To Do And How To Cope

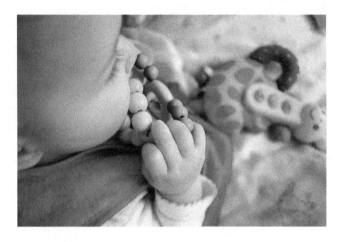

Most babies get forceful now and again. Fits of rage and destructive practices—hitting, kicking, scratching, and gnawing—don't mean you're a horrible parent—however, the source of inspiration.

In any event up to three, a forceful little youngster isn't "terrible" or defiant. They are attempting to reveal to you something and haven't yet built up the language aptitudes or passionate propensities to convey them successfully. Either that, or they don't feel you're tuning in to them, and viciousness is the best way to stand out enough to be noticed.

Causes Of Biting And Hitting Toddlers

Small kids may not understand that hitting can hurt because the sentiment of empathy doesn't wholly exist until around age. Regardless of whether your kid comprehends the thought, she may not contain herself; 1-year-olds have no motor control.

Their purposes behind hitting are blameless enough and, for the most part, can be categorized as one of these classifications.

She is attempting to impart. Like every other person, small kids get exhausted, ravenous, tired, and overpowered. The thing that matters is that they come up short on the verbal aptitudes to impart these feelings, making them much more baffled.

She is safeguarding her region. You have most likely seen your kid hitting all the more regularly on the play area or a play date. The explanation? She's encircled by a gathering of children who snatch his toys, push him down, or attack his space and don't listen when he says, "Stop!" Oh, mine! "Not acting out of resentment requires drive control, which kids don't wholly ace until they are more seasoned.

She is having an awful day. At the point when your kid is having a terrible day, you can lash out at her since she is crotchety and needs adapting abilities. "Indeed, even kids who don't hit or chomp can frequently lose control when pushed or toward the finish of a taxing day," says Dr. Schechter.

She is mimicking another person. Your kid may have seen his more seasoned sibling and companion hitting him, and now he needs to get in on the activity. "For certain youngsters, there is an experimentation factor," says parent counselor Jennifer Shu, M.D., a pediatrician in Atlanta. "They see another person hitting, and they think, 'Well, how about we see what that feels like.'"

She is volatile. A few youngsters, who are less quiet commonly, are inclined to lead with their clench hands or teeth. "A great deal comes to demeanor," clarifies the kid therapist Stanley Turecki, M.D., The Difficult Child creator. Though a few children shrug and move when somebody gets barney from their hands, others get into the fighting mode.

You are attempting new things. Little youngsters like to try circumstances and logical results: "If I do this current, what will occur?" They're merely utilizing the main assets they have, says Theodore Dix, Ph.D., partner educator of a human turn of events and family science at the University of Texas, Austin. "They don't be able to get what they need reasonably so they can be fierce or excessively troublesome," he says.

She needs her space. Little youngsters don't have away from different relations. They now and again end up cornered in a bit of room, excessively near other kids. Reflexively, they're attempting to strike (or hack or chomp) to leave.

How you react to your child's attack is the key to nipping it in the bud. Here is a general guideline: squat down to her level, look her in the eye and say in a calm, stern voice, "Don't hit. Hitting hurts." The excessive explanation is lost on the little ones and can backfire. The more your child gets involved in the discussion, the more attention she will get from being aggressive.

Reward Good Behavior

Instead of paying attention to your child only when she is misbehaving, congratulate her on being good whenever you can. For example, when you ask to swing on the swing instead of just pushing another child out of the way. Aim to give your child the most attention for positive behavior and reduce the time she spends on malicious behavior.

Praise him when he says what he wants, and be specific and honest with it ("Well done for asking for a chance!"). Also, remember to praise your efforts to do something, even if you can't do it. ("Well done for asking the girl if you could have a turn. I know she didn't answer and you were frustrated, right?") This helps your little one develop confidence and feel good about himself. Over time, you will realize how powerful words can be.

Utilize The Following Tactics To Deal With Undesirable Behavior:

1. Track violent conduct with legitimate results.

On the off chance that your youngster gets into the indoor play community's ball opening and starts tossing balls at different children, get her out. Sit with him and watch while other youngsters play. Clarify that you can return when you both feel like you are prepared to participate in the fun without harming anybody.

Make an effort not to dissuade your baby, for instance, by asking, "How might you like the ball to be tossed at you?"

Despite everything, small kids can't imagine another kid's perspective or change how they carry on dependent on reason. By and large, this intellectual development doesn't happen until kids are four or five years of age. Be that as it may, small kids can comprehend the outcomes.

2. Keep your temper

Shouting, hitting, or telling your kid that he is wicked won't change his conduct. He will turn out to be more aggravated and take in new things from you to attempt. In all actuality, watching you remain calm can be the initial phase in realizing how to oversee it.

3. Cutoff points are clear

Attempt to react quickly when your kid is forceful. Try not to hold up until she hits her sibling a third time. You should know soon when you accomplished something incorrectly. Attempt to talk decidedly with her ("The standard is thoughtful hands" or "Please utilize your inward voice"). Caution her that on the off chance that she continues hitting, she won't have the option to play with her sibling. If it doesn't stop, expel him from the circumstance for a moment or two. Clarify that what you did wasn't right. At that point, let him return.

4. Be predictable

At whatever point you can, respond to every scene as you did before. Your anticipated reaction ("The standard is delicate hands, recollect") will set up an example that your youngster will expect. In any event, when he's away and humiliated by his child's conduct, you don't lash out of disgrace. Keep in mind. Different guardians have additionally been there. On the off chance that individuals gaze, say, "Does anybody need a two-year-old?"

5. Instruct choices

Hold up until your kid has quieted down; at that point, talk smoothly about what occurred. Assist him with naming his feelings, tune in to what he is stating, and acknowledge his emotions, regardless of whether they are irate. Inquire as to whether you can clarify what annoyed you. Underline that it is normal to have furious sentiments, yet it isn't alright to show them by hitting, kicking, circling. Assist him with finding a superior method to react, maybe by discussing it ("Tommy, you're making me frantic") or approaching a grown-up for help.

6. Ask your youngster what the standard is

When he's lashed out, he'll most likely be glad to mention to you what the law is, regardless of whether he didn't tail it. Requesting that her recall the standard strengthens the conduct she expects, and this will steadily absorb. It might even be superior to ordering a (frequently questionable) expression of remorse.

7. Cutoff screen time

Kid's shows and different shows for little youngsters can be loaded up with shouting, undermining, in any event, pushing and hitting. Cut off the measure of screen time your minor child has and control what she sees, particularly if she is inclined to hate. A few rules suggest that kids age two and under don't have screen time.

On the off chance that you let your kid sit in front of the TV, and when you do, watch it with him and discussion about what he saw straightaway.

8. Help your youngster be dynamic

Except if your youngster gets an opportunity to consume her bountiful vitality, she may think that its a fear at home. Give her enough unstructured recess, ideally outside, paying little heed to the climate, to release pressure. The rules suggest that kids younger than five should be dynamic for in any event, three hours every day.

9. Support personal time

Notwithstanding being dynamic, it is likewise essential to urge your youngster to have rest, playing discreetly alone. Doing so implies that you find out how to invigorate your creative mind and have a good time without relying upon yourself. While whenever it can be a decent time, the advances from lunch to nap time, or supper to sleep, time is ideal.

10. Try not to be reluctant to look for help

Once ina whilee, violent conduct requires more intercession than guardians can give. On the off chance that your baby frequently carries on forcefully, irritates other youngsters, or if your endeavors to control her conduct have little impact, converse with your primary care physician. She may allude you to somebody that works in kid conduct.

Together, they can get to the base of the conduct and help your youngster get past it. Keep in mind. He is still exceptionally youthful. If you work with him quietly, his violent upheavals will, in all likelihood, be a relic of times gone by.

Manners

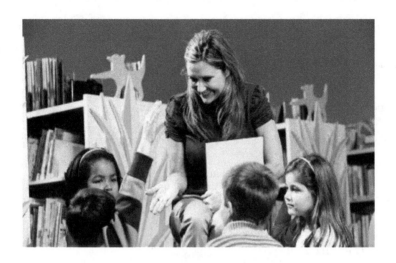

From a young age, children copy and mimic adults. They notice our every move and word. This is also true when it comes to manners. While children strive to please their parents and show quite pleasant temperaments, children between the ages of 2 and 6 are still mastering their abilities to reason and judge. Experts and researchers agree that the tantrums, that so famously give year two its nickname "the terrible twos," are a normal part of childhood.

In addition to the brain development that increases a child's ability to reason and judge between years 2 and 6, children also must acquire the vocabulary and ability to communicate. This can be a frustrating process, sometimes ending in tears.

However, this doesn't mean that manners can't be taught and learned during this time.

Children can be introduced to many lessons about manners that will help them develop excellent habits in this area for life. People skills and the ability to empathize with others, among other skills, will determine the success of your child's future relationships, personal and professional.

Teaching manners, people skills, and healthy ways of expressing emotions focus on the lessons included in this book. In the Montessori classroom, these are also referred to as "Grace and Courtesy" lessons. They are:

- Calming Down
- Being Thankful
- Saying "please"
- Saying "sorry."
- Resolving Conflict
- Being Silent

<u>Calming Down</u>

After an upset, it cannot be easy to achieve calm again. Many Montessori preschool classrooms dedicate a corner of the school known as the "peace corner." One of its various purposes is to provide a space to calm down.

Space often features some pillows, a carpet, a vase where the peace flower is kept, a calming picture, and rotating items that may include a stress ball, a sand timer, or a Zen garden. Here, children can regain their sense of calm after an upset.

You could quickly implement a similar space in your home. If you do decide to do so, it's best to include your child in the designing and preparing the area. This way, they will feel ownership over the corner and be more likely to care for and use it.

To create the space together, explain to your child that you will create a peaceful corner. Tell them that one of the purposes of the area will be to provide a place to be upset. In my experience, children can learn to use the space quite well, appreciating it as a short-term refuge when they are bitter. Children enjoy crying into the pillows, squeezing the stress ball, or raking sand patterns in the mini Zen garden.

Some other strategies for teaching calming down include taking deep, belly breathes, using a stress ball (you can make your own by filling a balloon with flour and then tying it off), or even hitting pillows. Each child may feel differently when angry or may have different responses for different kinds of upsets.

Choose a moment when your child is not upset to present one of the ideas. Practice the concept, and then, when your child is upset, invite him or her to practice one of the strategies. It may take a few upsets, but eventually, your child may want to try one approach.

Finally, remember that you are their model. What do you do to calm down when you're upset? That will probably be within their first responses. Try to match your reaction to what you'd like your child to do.

Being Thankful

Practicing thankfulness or gratefulness has been linked to health benefits and greater levels of happiness. Additionally, it builds and grows relationships, so it's beneficial for at least two groups.

It starts by teaching your child to say "thank you," and ensuring that your child frequently hears you say, "thank you." However, you can cultivate thankfulness in your child by engaging in some additional activities such as:

- Writing/coloring "thank you" cards
- Talking about what you enjoyed most about the day before bed
- Making baked goods and giving them away as "thank you" gifts for important people in your child's life (teachers, coaches, grandparents, etc.)

Saying "Please"

Like being thankful, saying "please" must be heard frequently to make its way quickly into your child's vocabulary and communication habits. Make a point of the importance of saying "please" by providing a lesson shared in many Montessori preschool classrooms.

If you have more than one child, you can do this activity with several of your children. If not, invite friends over or do this lesson as part of a play date. Plan a small snack such as popcorn or apple slices. Invite the children to sit in a circle.

Begin passing the plate or bowl around, allowing each child to take a few pieces of popcorn or an apple slice. Have one child hold the container while the neighbor asks, "May I please have a slice?" the child answers "yes," and the other says, "thank you."

Children can continue practicing the "please" and "thank you" game until the snack is gone.

Saying "Sorry"

Once again, modeling is one of the best ways to encourage your child to speak, "sorry." You can place additional emphasis on this by role-playing or talking through situations with your child.

For example, ask your child to play a game with you. Say, for instance, "Let's pretend I step on your foot." Proceed to "step" on your child's foot. Then, perform an exaggerated reaction of surprise and say, "I'm sorry." Ask your child to try. Then, talk about how, when you hurt someone else and feel bad about it, it's nice to say "I'm sorry."

Resolving Conflict

In many Montessori preschool classrooms, the peace corner is also a place to resolve conflict. It is here that the peace flower comes into play. This beautiful routine for resolving conflict helps children take turns talking and express their feelings. You can teach your child using the following steps.

1. Show your child the peace flower (can be a silk flower or real). Explain that it is very fragile, like our feelings.

2. Say that sometimes we get angry with each other or with our friends and that it's normal.

3. Tell your child that when they disagree, they can come to the peace corner.

4. Each person who disagrees has a turn to hold the peace flower. When holding it, they should keep it close to the heart, where we often feel our emotions.

5. The person who is holding the peace flower is allowed to talk. The other person listens.

6. The people who disagree take turns passing the flower back and forth until they can agree on a solution.

Providing a role-play of how this might work is often very helpful. If possible, give an example of the peace flower conflict resolution process with another adult. Among siblings and friends, this model can work well and can also be useful for parent-child disagreements.

Being Silent

Montessori believed that being silent and still was an essential skill for children. In the preschool, she taught children the "silence" game in which children tried to be very quiet for as long as possible. The game ends when the teacher whispers each child's name to line up at the door for the end of the day.

You can encourage your child to practice this art by sitting very still and trying to be silent. Ask your child to listen very carefully to see if they can hear breathing or any movement in their body at all. You may even want to time them to see how long they can last, and encourage them to be quiet for more extended periods.

Looking at it today, it seems that Montessori was encouraging a meditation of sorts. The silence game is a time of sitting at the moment, silently reflecting and simply being.

Many parents know that children often decide that they need or want attention at inopportune times. For example, when the phone rings or two adults are having a meaningful conversation. For children who are skilled in silence, a discussion about when silence should be used outside of its meditative purposes can help.

The more children are aware of, and the more explicit expectations are, the easier it is for them to comply and be respectful. Explain to your child that when you are on the phone or when two adults are talking, that they should practice silence unless there is an emergency. Then, ensure that you immediately attend to your child when you are finished so that their needs are also met.

Common Issues

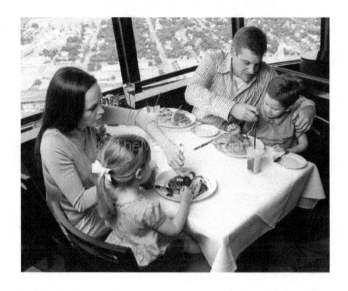

Parents and caregivers want to do what is best for their children. Still, if this were easy, there wouldn't be as many books, websites, and parenting theories devoted to helping parents and caregivers work out what's best for their toddlers and their families. Many areas are universally tough spots for parents and caregivers and their toddlers, and we will touch on them here.

Parent Perspective

There is an easy fix that has the potential to bring new levels of peace to parents and caregivers, and it requires a simple reframe: In any trying moment when toddler behavior seems to be in immediate need of correction and discipline, before asking how we should do that, first ask why is our toddler doing that? All behavior is communication, and all too often, we view toddler behavior through an adult frame of reference. We may watch a toddler teasing and taunting their infant sibling mercilessly and immediately jump to an assumption that they are being naughty and mean to them. If we instead take a moment and look into the behavior, why we may find something more there. For instance, has the toddler been struggling with their new role as an older sibling? Has their recently been a new development that made them feel like they were giving something up, perhaps an old beloved baby toy that has now been handed down to the baby despite their protests to keep it for themselves? Does the toddler now find themselves having to fight for their parent's attention? The answers to these questions will shed light on the true why of the behavior. All parents and caregivers develop an individualized response that can accurately address the root issue, rather than placing a short-term band-aid type solution. In this scenario, it sounds like rather than just removing the toddler from access to baby (which is the easy answer here), it will also be necessary for parents and caregivers to ensure that the toddler feels loved and secure in their place in the family, as a new baby always creates new dynamics that can sometimes make little ones feel displaced.

Always begin with the why before the what to do.

The 'S' Word

The 'S' word is enough to strike confusion into any toddler's heart during a playdate: Share!

Unfortunately, parents and caregivers often contribute to the confusion and frustration with the notion of sharing because they often attempt to teach sharing by forcing sharing. It usually looks something like this: Toddler one has a toy. Toddler two toddles over and looks longingly at the toy. Toddler two reaches out for the toy. Toddler one pulls the toy back. Toddler two makes a frustrated noise as they reach out for the toy again. Now parent/caregiver of toddler one notices and attempts to teach what they consider to be a valuable lesson and tells toddler one, "share!" while taking the toy out of toddler one's hands and placing it into toddler two's hands. Toddler one erupts into tears.

In this particular scenario, what did the toddlers learn? Toddler learned that to "share" means that someone will come and take the thing you are using out of your hands and give it to someone else. Toddler two learned that to "share" means that you want something, so someone else will come and get it for you. Neither toddler understands a bit about what it means to share.

To begin with, let's consider what sharing means. Sharing is the ability to give some of whatever you have to another in a spirit of generosity. Sharing is not having something taken from you or being coerced into giving it. Can you imagine if you were standing at the park in a group of friends when suddenly one of them reaches out for the keys to your car, demanding that you "share"? And then, when you react by pulling your car keys away, another friend that is bigger than you pull them out of your hand and gives them to the other friend, reminding you that it's nice to "share." This would be theft, not sharing!

It is the same thing we do with our small children. Sharing is a developmental skill that comes naturally after they have seen it modeled it before them enough times. Even then, sharing is not always a natural choice for small children to make, which is developmentally appropriate. It can be challenging for parents and caregivers to sit back and watch as their toddler pulls back a toy that another toddler wants. Still, if parents and caregivers can put their feelings of discomfort aside, they might realize that toddlers are learning critical social skills in their song and dance of "I want but can't have" and "I have and won't give." When parents and caregivers step in to 'help,' it takes the opportunity for them to get their bearings and make the required connections away from them.

Sharing is a skill that is learned over time, not forced.

Separation Anxiety

Some toddlers find themselves very anxious when separated from their parents and primary caregivers. Still, it is often due to how parents and caregivers separate rather than the actual act of separation. Two extremes often occur when parents and caregivers are separating from toddlers: On one end of the spectrum, parents and caregivers usually try to sneak out and away from their toddler without them realizing it, assuming that if they avoid any tear-filled goodbyes, then there will be no stress and anxiety surrounding their absence. The other end of the spectrum is when parents and caregivers spend too long saying their goodbyes and return for extra hugs and kisses at the slightest whimper.

The disappearing act is not fooling anybody. It can increase anxiety and agitation in toddlers because not only is their parent/caregiver gone from them, but they are gone without a trace! There is no warning, no explanation, just here one second and gone the next. This is incredibly disrespectful to children and assumes that it is better to leave them hanging in confusion than to deal with their big emotions during goodbyes. There is no need for this.

The long and drawn-out goodbye is responsible for making many a toddler wonder, "if my parent can't seem to let me go, then there must be a reason for it. I must not be safe without them." Toddlers look to their parents and caregivers to be healthy, confident leaders. As such, parents and caregivers must project confidence in their toddlers, so they know they are safe, secure, and taken care of. The way to impart this message while leaving is to keep an upbeat, steady voice during the goodbye, and tell your toddler you are leaving. "Mommy is going to work now, but I love you and will see you very soon! Have fun today." As you say this, kisses and hugs can be exchanged and then step back and confidently move towards the door. The moment the parent falters and looks around with uncertainty, the toddler recognizes this as a signal that perhaps they are not safe and will not be well taken care of. This does an incredible disservice to the toddler.

Calm and Confident Leader

So much of disciplining toddlers lovingly and respectfully depends on this energy: a calm and confident leader. Toddlers look to their parents and caregivers for cues on how they should proceed in the world, and modeling is the most effective way to show them what is expected of them.

In all of your interactions with your toddler moving forward, remember this. You can and should respectfully acknowledge their fears, frustrations, issues, and upsets, but you should do this as a calm and confident leader. In doing so, you set the tone for both their success and yours.

Practical Application

Now that you are armed with knowledge and the techniques of effective discipline, it is time to learn their application. Having experience of effectively disciplining your toddler is helpful, so you will know how to respond appropriately in situations where your toddler tends to misbehave. Take note that punishing a child takes self-control, perseverance, and even practice.

The following are based on real-life case studies. First, read the situation and then think of a solution. After this, look at the recommended solution, so you will know how your decision matches with the suggested action. Take note that the answers below are merely guided and do not claim to be the best course of action in every situation. After all, the art of discipline is a continuously developing system.

Charles Knocked Over The Building Blocks Of His Sister, Nina.

Should you scold Charles, lock him up in his room, or maybe ignore it? After all, it was just a toy that he knocked down. What should you tell Charles?

Solution: Tell Charles not to do it again and apologize to his sister by helping her rebuild the building blocks.

While Playing A Game, Marco Keeps Throwing The Clay Around.

Should you end the game right away and tell him to clean his mess? Should you let him enjoy what he is doing and continue to scatter clay all about the place? What should you tell Marco?

Solution: Tell Marco to "keep the clay on the table so that we can keep playing."

Max Is Riding The Bike And Would Not Let His Friend, Sarah, To Have A Turn.

Should you encourage Max not to share his bike with his friend, Sarah? Would you tell Max to stop riding the bike right away and embarrass him in front of his friend?

Solution: Tell Max to take two or three more turns, and then let his friend turn.

Nicole And Her Friend, Jenna, Were Playing With The Dolls. Nicole Forcefully Took The Beauty That Jenna Was Playing With.

What should you tell Nicole?

Solution: Tell Nicole that it is Jenna's turn to play with the doll and that if she (Nicole) wants to play with it, she should tell Jenna, "Jenna, may I have a turn to play with the doll?"

Max And Peter Were Running Outside. Max Pushed Peter.

Should you tell your kid, Max, to stop playing right away? Should you wait for an explanation before you respond?

Solution: Tell Max, "Max, you hurt Peter. Apologize and tell him you will not push him again."

Instead Of Stacking His Blocks, Your Toddler Starts Throwing Them.

Should you tell your kid not to play with the blocks anymore? Can you ask him to stop what he is doing?

Solution: Say, "The blocks are for stacking."

You Saw Your Child Swearing At His Friend. After A Few Minutes, He Approached You And Explained What Happened.

Should you have him grounded? How can you explain to him in simple terms that swearing is bad? Would it be acceptable to get angry at your child for severe such misbehavior?

Solution: Tell you to toddle that swearing is not a pleasant and happy word and that he should never say that word to anyone. Also, reassure him that you understand him and that you are on his side, but stress the lesson that he should not swear again no matter the reason.

Your Child Starts Breaking His Toy.

Is it a good idea to stop buying him toys? Should you be mad at him?

Solution: Tell him that "You must be nice to your toys. Tell me you will not break your toys again."

Your Child, Frank, Punched His Friend.

Should you tell Frank to get inside the house and ground him for a day or even a week?

Solution: Take your kid, Frank, out to the side, and explain to him that it hurts when we get punched, especially by a friend. Tell him to apologize to his friend and say that he will not hit him again.

Your Child Starts To Draw On The Table With Colored Pens.

What should you tell your child?

Solution: Tell her to "Draw on the paper." Could you not make a big deal about it? You can also use the logical consequence technique and tell him to erase his drawing on the table and clean up his mess.

Your Kid Invites His Friend At Home. They Play The Computer. Your Kid Has Been Playing For A Long Time And Would Not Like To Share Anymore.

What should you tell your child?

Solution: Say, "Two more mouse clicks, and then, it is your friend's turn.

There Is A Party At Your Place. Your Child Is Shy To Be With A Large Group Of People And Runs Away Into Her Room Whenever You Try To Bring Him To Join Everyone.

Should you just let her stay in her room simply because she is shy?

Solution: Gently tell your child that she looks beautiful. Tell her that she can go to the large group all by herself after some time or hold your hand now and walk over to join everyone and enjoy the party.

You Receive A Note From His Teacher Saying That Your Child Is Disobedient. Your Child Says That It Is Not True And That Everybody Hates That Teacher.

Should you ignore the letter from the teacher?

Solution: Tell your child that "In school, we need to mind the teachers. I always listened to my teachers when I was in preschool. I will schedule a meeting with your teacher."

While Playing With The Building Blocks, Your Toddler Took His Sister's Toy Without Asking For Permission, And He Is Not Willing To Give It Back.

What should you tell your toddler?

Solution: Tell him, "Your sister was playing with that block. Give it back to her, and let us find some blocks for you."

During A Family Game, John Starts Hitting His Sister, Melissa.

What should you do?

Solution: Tell him calmly to keep his hands to himself and apologize to his sister, or he will have to sit out of the family activity.

After Playing A Game With Your Toddler, She Does Not Want To Help In Cleaning The Mess.

Should you force your kid to clean up? Should you be upset with her?

Solution: Tell your toddler that the mess was because of the game. If she still wants to play a game with you next time, she should help you clean up the area.

During A Family Activity, Your Toddler Begins Speaking Out Loud And Would Not Sit Still While You Are Talking, Which Also Disrupts The Activity.

What should you tell your kid?

Solution: Tell him that everyone has a chance to talk and wait for his turn. Also, tell him that he will have to sit still; otherwise, the family activity can no longer be continued.

During A Family Reunion, Your Child Does Not Want To Join Everyone At The Table For Dinner.

Should you grab your child's arm and force her to join everyone?

Solution: Tell her that it is time for dinner. You can also add, "Do you want to go by yourself or hold my hand?"

Samantha Is Building A Tower With Her Blocks, But Liza Keeps Knocking It Down. Samantha Is Now Getting Frustrated.

What should you tell Liza?

Solution: Tell her to apologize and leave Samantha's tower alone, and then offer to help her build her outlook.

Your Toddler, Stella, Refuses To Eat Her Snack.

What should you tell her?

Solution: Tell her to finish her snack, or she can start doing her homework.

Marie Is Dancing On A Chair, And You Are Worried That She Might Fall.

Would you explain to Marie the risks of dancing on a chair?

Solution: Say, "Marie, put your feet on the floor."

Gabriel Is Yelling At His Friend.

What should you do?

Solution: Take Gabriel aside, and then tell him that he must talk nicely to continue playing.

Rose Is Dancing In The Room When It Is Time For Her To Sit Down And Read.

What should you tell her?

Solution: "Rose, it is time to read. Which book do you want me to read to you?"

It Is Time To Go Home, But Your Child Still Wants To Play Outside.

How can you convince your child to go home?

Solution: Say, "It is time to go home. Shall we race to the door?"

As you can see, it is not challenging to discipline as a toddler as long as you are ready. There is also no need to use any form of physical. Discipline is made in a kind and calm manner. Words, as long as you use the correct words, and say them correctly, are powerful.

Being able to teach your toddler good manners and right conduct is always possible. It is never too late for a change. Every time your toddler tries your patience, it is a sign that there is a learning opportunity that you can take advantage of.

When disciplining your toddler, always focus on building a positive relationship. Of course, this does not mean that you have to sacrifice your authority as a parent. Filial love requires sincerity, perseverance, a fair amount of patience, continuing support, and undying love for your child. Last but not least, remember that children are very fragile. You should be careful with their heart.

After The Tantrum Do's And Don'ts

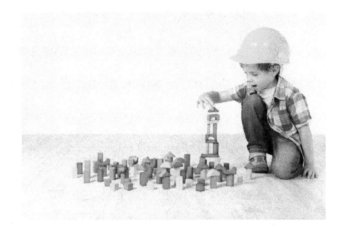

Finally, we are going to look over what to expect when a tantrum has concluded. No one likes dealing with tantrums, and when it does happen, people are generally hopeful that they can avoid more in the future. Unfortunately, there will almost always be another tantrum at some point. However, the way you handle the aftermath of the temper can help you learn how to recognize what has happened and how to begin to move on from it altogether.

In particular, you may find that your child is quite upset or ashamed after the tantrum. Remember, for most children. It is a matter of their emotions going haywire—they are not trying to misbehave. Children want to please their parents, and they will do whatever they can to do so. If you make your child feel like they have failed to do so, they will feel bad.

With that in mind, let's go over what not to do after a tantrum. These should be avoided—after all, you should be treating your child with the tact and grace that he or she deserves. Your child is not trying to give you a hard time. Yes, that point has been reiterated throughout the book—because it is true. Your child is having a hard time but is not trying to give you a hard time intentionally. Remember that when you approach the situation and allow it to color your response.

- Don't shame: Your child is probably already feeling entirely wrong about the outburst, and piling onto that is not going to help. Children are smart—he or she already knows that there was some problem with the behaviors, and that is enough. Ensure that you do not tell your child that they messed up or try to make your child feel bad about it.

- Don't call your child bad: No children are naughty. They may be bad at self-regulating, but they are not bidding themselves. Remember to avoid labeling the child themselves and instead focus on marking the behaviors. This means there should be no asking a child why they are so bad.

- Don't make the punishment last all day: Make sure that after a tantrum and after you have gone over the problem with your child, you return to how things were before. It would help if you did not treat your child differently for the day because of their tantrum, as this is only causing more problems for them.

- Don't withhold affection: You should never use your love as a punishment. Do not withhold your liking from your child. That is a basic need in those tender years, and withholding it will only cause hurt. Your child trusts you to be their safe spot, and if you take that away from them, how are they supposed to respond?

Beyond just what not to do, however, there is a way that you can deal with tantrums after the fact. When the emotions have calmed down, you can turn everything into a learning experience for your child. Remember, your child is still developing. Your child is still learning how he or she can navigate the world, which is no easy feat. It takes years and years to get all of those social nuances down, and you should not fault your child for not being able to manage their feelings when many adults still struggle to do so long after childhood. Being a child is challenging, and you need to remember to have that compassion for your child, so they do not feel like they will be a failure. Make sure that you do treat your child with that compassion and do the following after the tantrum. In doing so, you can take it from a moment of anger and frustration and help it mold into a healing and learning experience. With that in mind, consider doing the following after a tantrum has subsided:

- Do talk about it: When the temper is over, and your child can stop and think, it is time to have a friendly, age-appropriate conversation about what has happened. You can do this in many different ways. For example, you could talk to your child about how he or she has done something that is not a nice thing. Remember that wording matters here—you tell the child that the behavior was not friendly, not that your child was not lovely. While you may be able to differentiate between the two, your child cannot. Your child will not understand the nuance between them behaving a certain way and being a certain way. Spend time talking about what went wrong.

- Ask what they can do next time: Make sure that after the talk, you ask your child how they may respond better in the future. Younger kids may not be able to articulate this, but older toddlers and preschoolers usually can. They do not have to go into extreme detail—all they have to do is tell you how they can change up what they were doing to better cope with the future situation.

- Encourage healthy and proper apologies: Remember, this is a learning experience. Your child has done something wrong that has upset someone, whether that was you or someone else. With that in mind, you must be able to encourage your child to understand how apologies work. Apologies happen everywhere, and because of that, you must be able to remind your child how to do so appropriately. Remember to encourage an apology that includes "I'm sorry for doing [insert behavior here]." You want them to understand what it was that they did that was a problem, why it was a problem, and that the other person saw it as a problem. This is the manner that everyone should apologize—it acknowledges fault and what had happened.

- Hug: When you are done talking, and the apology is over, you should always make it a point to hug your child. This reminds your child that you do love him or her—it tells your child that, no matter what happens, you are still there and that you are always going to love them. You do not want them to assume that your love is conditional—something that can lead to all sorts of problems later on in life. Your pet should be freely given, and you should remind your child that it is there shortly after your child is done with the tantrum.

15 Tips To Unleash The Child's Creative Potential

In this part, the tips are based on the recommendations of renowned French psychologist and psychologist Michèle Freud. These tips help to unleash the creative potential of every child.

1. Support Total Freedom

Creativity is expressed when it is not repressed. Give the child total freedom to express himself/herself. Let the child pursue interests instead of forcing him/her to sit down and finish tasks that do not cater to their needs.

One of the most critical mistakes is limiting the child's interest. Many parents mean well when they try hard to mold their child into their concept of who he/she should be.

For example, parents often smother their child's creativity when they force them to memorize flags and country capitals. Sure, it may seem impressive for a three-year-old to know all the flags and means, even all the train stops in a faraway foreign country. However, if the child isn't interested, all that hard work will be a colossal waste. Worse, the child's potential can be seriously hampered by the hostile environment fostered by a forced activity.

2. Encourage Personal Expression

A child must have an active role in choosing what activity to pursue. Parents only work by introducing options. The child ultimately decides.

For example, parents can show the child how to play with a xylophone, drums, keyboards, guitar, and violin. Choices shouldn't stop there. They should also offer other objects such as a ball, building blocks, construction playsets, music to dance to or sing along with, paints, dolls, and so on. The more choices the child has, the greater the opportunities for expression and exploration of creative potential.

3. Do Not Judge The Quality Of Results. Appreciate The Child Whatever The Results

Creativity is all about creating. It is not about reproducing what is already existing.

With these concepts in mind, parents and teachers should not judge a child's results based on the work of others. The child's painting should be appreciated as it is and not compared to how another child used better colors and techniques.

Teachers and parents should also remember that a child's creative expression is precisely that – an indication of how he/she sees the world or experience the activity. It is not about having a child to play Mozart exceptionally well but more about the child expressing himself/herself through music.

4. Recognize And Support Emotional Sensitivity

Children naturally fear anything new, as adults feel the same, too. It is a normal reaction to something unknown. Adults can help children feel more confident by explaining what to expect with an activity. Fear is significantly reduced when a person or a child knows what to expect.

Teach the child to verbalize fear. This also helps deal with emotions. Verbalizing can start by letting the child describe what he/she feels. Teach the child to give a name to that feeling. This way, the unseen surface starts to take on a form through that name. The child is then abler to handle it because it has an image he/she has created for that feeling. Something known is more comfortable to hold than something faceless, nameless, and entirely unknown.

5. Support Development Of The Senses

Teaching and educating a child is more than just chanting letters and numbers, memorizing tables, and recognizing colors and shapes. Education should also be a means for a child to unleash creative potential. For this to happen, a child has to have a variety of sensory experiences.

These experiences cater to their development level. Young children are at a stage where they are starting to discover many things in their environment and their bodies. This period of discovery can be taken advantage of to help children develop and fine-tune their skills as well as discover and enhance their creative potential.

6. Provide Freedom For Creativity

Safety is a primary consideration. However, do not overdo it. According to Michèle Freud, it is not ideal to confine children in too-safe spaces with items designed especially for them. This kind of environment produces a monotony.

Remember, again, that children are at a point in their lives where everything is new and ready to be discovered. At this stage, the child has to be exposed to a variety of objects to find, learn, and be creative. Monotony kills the child's initiative to discover and create. Even adults get bored with the same things every day.

7. More On "Real" Toys Than "Educational Games."

Educational games have become a go-to for many parents. They think that these are the best toys they can give their children to raise them smart and creative.

According to Michèle Freud, educational toys are not exactly what parents expect them to be. These educational toys can hamper creative potential. These toys were designed to be used in specific ways only. That leaves very little room for individuality. Once the child has discovered how the education toy works, there's nothing else to do with it. There is no room for creativity. There are no opportunities to find new ways to use the objects.

8. Give Importance To Artistic Activities

Many caregivers and parents try to avoid artistic activities such as painting. They also put less emphasis on art education. They'd instead expose their children to educational toys or educational apps on tablets. They like their children to memorize capitals and train stops and flags or learn addition at a very early age.

Art feeds creativity. It lets children know that there are many forms to express creative potential. It can be through music, dance, painting, photography, sculptures, and so on. Art is a world full of possibilities- something that a child should learn at an early age.

9. Allow Originality In Many Forms.

Let the child be original. Creativity thrives in originality, not in mimicking others. Simple things that a child is allowed to choose for himself/herself can already have a significant impact on his/her self-esteem and creativity.

This can be as simple as allowing a child to choose the clothes to wear. If a child wants to wear a tiara and pirate dress, then so be it. If the child wants to use rubber boots to school, then let him. If a child wants to wear one red sock and a yellow one, why not?

There's no danger in dressing in something you want.

10. Respect Divergent Thinking

Children do not know how to distinguish reality from fiction properly. They think that fairies are real and that their teacher can teach ogres manners. They believe that what happens in the cartoons they watched can also occur in real life. They think that the lion at the zoo knows Simba from The Lion King.

This fluidity of thinking between fantasy and reality allows children to shift from one idea to the next, from one interest to another rapidly. This, surprisingly, also will enable children to become more creative thinkers.

Child experts call this "divergent thought." This is a unique event in children that should be allowed to flourish during this period in their development. It's an event uniquely fantastic in the younger years. It should be taken advantage of to facilitate the development of creative potential.

11. Get Involved With Nature

Child researchers and psychoanalysts found that children ages 4 to 7 have an increased interest in nature. This is a period where activities that allow them to work with and, in essence, is best. Bring them outside to run and play, touch the grass, feel the wind and sun on their skin, play with rocks, or gather flowers. Bring them to the beach or the park.

Swim in the sea or wade in the river. Take them for a walk in the woods. Go camping or fishing.

If possible, let the child have a pet. If not, have a plan for the child to take care of.

All these activities not only cater to their interests. These also instill valuable lessons they bring them into adulthood.

12. Include Children In Cooking Activities

Food is an excellent way to teach children in a fun, engaging way. Michèle Freud advises parents and educators to allow children to work with food. This is also one of the vital Montessori activities. Food prep will enable children to work with various textures of materials, as well as learn how to use multiple tools. All these help them to learn motor skills, discrimination, and a few math concepts. Children, according to Michèle Freud, should even be allowed to create their recipes. This way, they can experiment with taste, smell, and textures. They can; earn countless things by just letting them mess around in the kitchen.

13. Stimulate Imagination

Children love to listen to stories. They also love to tell stories of their own. Give opportunities for the child to tell their own stories to encourage their imagination. This is an excellent exercise to promote more areas for expression of creativity.

Some parents are not keen on letting their children tell stories. They think that this will encourage the child to live in the fantasy world instead of becoming more grounded in reality. When the child starts to tell stories or show imagination, the parents immediately discourage it.

Parents should understand that children cannot relate to events in the same way that adults do.

Let the child develop his/her imagination. One way to do that is to encourage storytelling.

14. Nourish Musical Sensibility

Music is also an effective way to unleash creative potential. How many geniuses have created their groundbreaking ideas with music in the background? How many artists have completed notable works of art while listening to music?

Music is a universal language that binds people from all walks of life and of all ages. It can help stimulate creativity in children, too. A study even found that certain types of music can help in promoting divergent thinking. That means increasing creativity. The study found that people who were exposed to music that evoked a happy feeling were able to come up with more ideas, most of which are innovative and creative compared to those who did not listen to music.

15. Support The "Builder" Spirit

Children are inclined to build something. A baby will start to put blocks on top of each other. Toddlers can start putting random things together and call them something. Older children build objects from clay or other art materials.

Provide building materials to enhance creativity and imagination. Take note that building activities should allow children to express their creativity, not to reproduce something they have seen or what the parent or teacher wants. The experience, the process counts more than the actual results. If a child builds a lopsided tower with two bases and calls it the Eiffel Tower, respect that outcome. Do not point out what's wrong with the building and how it does not resemble the real Eiffel Tower. It is how the child wants to represent the Eiffel Tower as he/she sees it or maybe wants it to look like. Accept it and recognize this as a creative expression.

The Listening Process

To understand your listening behavior and increase your active listening skills, you will learn about the listening process. Don't be afraid! A little theory will help you to understand listening and give you the knowledge to apply it to your interactions.

There are several stages involved in the process of listening. Despite being distinct phases, they happen almost simultaneously as you look. They are, in brief, as follows:

Receiving- This is the physical function of hearing, where you receive the actual sound as vibrations in your ear, and transmitted to your brain. Besides audio, any visual cues such as body language and eye contact will also be picked up on.

Attending- When the message has received, i.e., physically picked up on by your senses and carried to your brain, it must then participate. At this stage, it is your job to pay attention to the message by holding it firmly in short-term memory (Baddley & Hitch, 1974). The more engagement you pay to the speaker's signals at this stage, the more likely you are of taking in what communicated. It is essential in active listening to pay close attention to the speaker because without doing so, and it is impossible to interpret and respond to what is said.

Perceiving- as the amount of attention you pay to the speaker, your perceptions are also a part of the listening process. This may sound unusual at first, but your background, experiences, beliefs, and your state of mind at the time, will all affect the message that you eventually receive. In short, you hear what you want to hear, or sometimes what you expect to hear. This is one reason why two people may listen to a different message from the same speaker; their perceptual filters have screened out or amplified other parts of the word.

You must have a perceptual filter. There are so many potential incoming signals in the world that it would simply blow your mind to take them all in. This can even be seen in essential functions like crossing the road, where you will notice (if you try to catch) that you will be more attuned to the noise of cars, speed, and distance, and to move at that moment. You may also blank out a lot of what else is around until you have made it to the other side.

Interpreting- So far on the journey, you have picked up the speaker's communication with your senses, which have carried it to the brain. You have held your attention on it for long enough that you have remembered it, and your perceptions have meanwhile done a great job of filtering out what is not needed, or what is in too severe a conflict with your conceptual outlook. Now, communication will be processed for meaning.

Your brain does this by attempting to fit the message into the correct linguistic categories, where it can discern for meaning according to your past experiences, thoughts and beliefs, and long-term memory. Linguistic groups are a technical term for how we break down in laypeople to categorize it, and if needed, analyze it.

In layman's terms, this means that you interpret and possibly an analysis of what has said. Your speaker's yourself at this point what understanding you can take from the speaker's message, and what the meaning is. Often the original meaning can be distorted, and can even end up completely different from what meant initially been.

One of the main aims of active listening is that it aims to understand what was meant by the speaker, rather than assuming our interpretation is correct.

Responding- The final stage of the listening process is the response. Internally, you are moving the message from short term to long term memory, if you need to retrieve it at a later point. The external response is given in the form of feedback, which may be an agreement, a reiteration or paraphrase, or a question regarding the message. The answer is an essential part of listening. Research by Leavitt and Mueller (1968) showed that the listener and speaker both gain confidence that the message has been understood. Both experience a high degree of satisfaction in conversation when feedback is given. This is something that active listening places a lot of emphasis on, and will be covered in more detail later on in the book. A response can go beyond feedback and can represent a transition between listening and speaking.

<u>Chinese Whispers</u>

You may be a little bogged down after that, but you must be familiar with the listening process; it provides a solid foundation for everything that is to come. You can now consider the above method of listening in the context of a game of Chinese whispers.

If you are not familiar with the game, Chinese whispers played in a group, who sit on a circle. Someone picked to start the game by coming up with a message to pass on to the person next to them. They think of a word and whisper it in the next person's ear, and it passed all the way around. The last person in the circle shouts the message out loud, and the original speaker reveals the original message. Then everyone laughs at how much the world has changed, and tries to work out where" the distortions occurred.

So, where do the distortions occur" How do" "My uncle packed sandwiches for all of us to take t" the beach," become "Try walking up this way to get to get to the sweets."?

Well, the distortions could occur at any point during the communication, and the more people the message goes around, the more distorted it is likely to become.

It could be a lack of attention and only part of the message received by someone. It could be that the message has been screened out by bias or misinterpreted by the impressions of someone. If the idea is emotionally charged or opinionated, then this is even more likely.

If you have not played this game yet, then consider getting it together to see how flawed our listening can be, even when the message is simple.

Why Is It Helpful To Understand This Process?

It is easy to see from studying the listening process described above that listening is a somewhat complicated pro" involves "multiple aspects. Instead of merely labeling yourself as a "bad listener," you can begin to understand what you can improve upon, or what stage of the listening process might be causing you to miss what is going on in the communication.

Do you pay enough attention to what is said? Is there a reason for you not doing? Are there too many actions in the room? Maybe you block out the real message because you don't want to hear it; it could be your perceptual filter, which causes you to cross wires with your loved ones. You could be misinterpreting the message that your friend is expressing. You may not be providing enough feedback for the speaker, who is relying on your response to engage in the conversation.

By understanding the whole process of listening, you can begin to see it differently. You can start to understand it.

A Positive Listening Attitude

Just in case your mind has been blown by the theory covered so far, you will be glad to know the tension will be momentarily released, and some simple advice offered to all of you. All of the steps of the process above can easily enhance with a positive listening attitude.

A positive listening attitude is to be interested in what is said. It varies across the conversation, and genuine interest rises and falls depending on your concern for the message. But being genuinely interested in what people have to say, and being open-minded towards new perspectives, helps you to function smoothly as a listener. Where your loved ones are concerned, you should always be interested.

Seeing listening as an active role in interaction also helps to cultivate this attitude. As a listener, it is your job to facilitate conversation. Please begin to see listening for the shining grace that it is; it is a valuable skill, and it helps people feel relaxed in their relationships with you.

Start to enjoy listening; be upbeat open-minded. "What Is an Active Listener?

You may have seen the words "active listener" mentioned several times in this book already; you may have also seen it mentioned elsewhere.

In Western culture, we often listen in a somewhat passive way; we wait for our turn while the other person speaks. We keep quiet out of respect for their message. Often, we are waiting for our turn again.

The active listener is engaged. They are as much a part of the conversation as the speaker because they see themselves as being partially responsible for the communication. They have a positive attitude towards listening; they are consciously working out what the message means, what angle the speaker is approaching, and their response. An active listener gives full attention to the conversation and is interested in what is said, why it is said, and how it can be encouraged.

CONCLUSION

Thank you for reading all this book!

Learning how to negotiate with your child is most beneficial. Thanks to that, they won't subconsciously feel they could do the way they want. They won't get the impression they're always under control and pressure, and their life is a band of constant bans.

Doing so will allow them to reinforce self-esteem and self-discipline within. As a result, they will also be able to assess their behavior and learn to make responsible decisions and consider the views of other family members.

Discipline and children have always been a contentious issue. Some still believe children should be seen and not heard, while others believe in free parenting, allowing their children unfettered access to the world around them. Nonetheless, every parent is different, and you'll need to adopt the approach that suits you the most.

A parent usually wants the best for their child; this is to help them grow into well-adjusted adults.

Remain calm when dealing with your toddler. This may not always be possible, but it's a goal to which you should try to adhere.

Remember that your child will mimic your actions. They are generally happiest when they make you satisfied, but toddlers find it very difficult to deal with frustration. They will not always be aware of whether their actions are right or wrong, and this is for you to teach them.

Discipline does not necessarily mean punishment. There have been many studies conducted which show toddlers and children respond better to positive measures than they do to negative ones. Praise and acknowledgment will always get better responses than shouting or fear.

Every parent seeks to provide their toddler with a happy and safe environment to play in and grow. To ensure this is possible, you should use the guidelines to establish discipline supplied within this book. With a little personal adaption, you'll find yourself with a happy child, which will ensure that you have a happy family, and they have the best possible start in life.

You have already taken a step towards your improvement.
Best wishes!

Potty Training

The Last Positive Parenting Guide to Potty Training. Toddler Discipline Tips and Tricks for Happy Kids and Peaceful Parents

Written By

Jennifer Siegel

Table of Contents

INTRODUCTION

Thank you for purchasing this book!

Potty Training Checklist

The truth is that parents must be careful not to lose their tempers with potty training because some kids aren't ready (Des Jarlais & Young, 2018). Ease up on the reins if you notice that your child isn't developmentally ready for its task because it causes tantrums that make you wish you waited.

A child must be able to run or walk steadily and urinate the right amount at once before you begin. Children of its age don't always 'wee' bucket loads, even if the parent changing the diaper seems to think so. Their bowel movements should also be predictable time-wise, and they should experience dry spells for about two hours at a time. These signs let you know that your toddler's motor development is ready.

Behavioral signs include being able to sit still for two to five minutes and pulling their undies up and down. You can't lose patience with a child who can't even drewqss themselves yet. Ready toddlers feel uneasy with wet diapers and often grunt or make noise when they have a bowel movement. Potty training isn't only about independence, but your child must also be proud of her accomplishments. Behavioral readiness exudes when a child stops resisting or being negative about potty training. Co-operation doesn't only make things easier, but it also tells you that your kid wants to learn. Resistance isn't always about discipline.

Cognitive or intellectual development also progress before you can gently guide your child to potty training. Can they understand instructions like "sit on the potty" or "time to pee?" Do they have words for poop and pee? A child must also understand where things belong in their bedroom to understand that poop doesn't belong in the diaper anymore. Kids who haven't developed a readiness don't know what their bodies are telling them. Finally, consider your child's attention span before you try to coach them gently with potty training.

Is their attention span long enough to get to the bathroom from the time they think they need to pee? Potty training discipline can be as simple as rhyming and turning the toilet into a fun space, but if you force your child to try to potty before they're ready, you fail. Look out for the various developmental milestones they need to achieve before using positive guidance, affectionate understanding, and considerate reassurance to teach them. There's a good chance that your child shows readiness by saying something when they see you go to the toilet.

"Mommy, diapers are yucky. We use the potty now?" One of my toddlers did precisely it. I was startled beyond belief, but I said: "Sure, honey. Let's use the potty."

Enjoy your reading!

10

Before You Begin

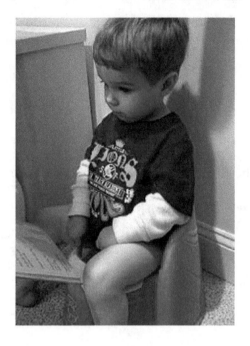

<u>What Is The Best Age For Toilet Training?</u>

What is the right age to train the bathroom? The response depends on you, your priorities, and the characteristics of your child.

What the scientific evidence says about the time of toilet training

- Infant toilet training (0-12 months)

- Older Infant / Toddler Training (12-18 months)

- Older children (18-24 months)

- Potty training after 24 months

The circumstance is altogether different in the United States, where kids can wear diapers for 2, 3, or even four years. As indicated by an ongoing report, African American guardians accept that potty preparing should begin around the year and a half by and large.

These perspectives are new. In the past ages, most American kids had no diapers by year and a half. Today, numerous kids don't ace the essential potty preparing abilities until they are right around three years of age. In an ongoing report, the more significant part of youngsters matured more than 32 months couldn't remain dry during the day. It is a pattern additionally saw in Europe. Since World War II, it takes youngsters longer and longer to learn potty abilities.

It shows that a prior period of potty preparation is secure. However, numerous guardians are stressed that underlying preparing can be impeding. They have heard "specialists" go to the washroom notice that early preparing messes conduct up or character issues. Accordingly, it is fantastic to find that these worries are strange.

The hour of latrine preparing: logical proof

Despite what you have caught wind of conduct issues or Freudian character issues, there is no logical proof that latrine preparation hurt the kids at a young age.

Early preparation can be helpful.

Notwithstanding forestalling diaper rash and diaper diseases, little youngsters who have been prepared in adolescence are more reluctant to have intermittent urinary lot contaminations.

Youngsters who don't begin preparing until the following two years may not arrive at its achievement until their third birthday celebration. There is additional proof that early students have a lower danger of creating incontinence issues sometime down the road.

For what reason does early preparing have horrible notoriety? One explanation is that individuals, in general, confound "when to prepare" with "how to prepare." Numerous individuals accept that early readiness requires the utilization of unpleasant and coercive techniques. It isn't so much that way. At the point when guardians utilize delicate, age-fitting methodologies, starting potty preparing is brilliant.

In any case, early planning isn't reasonable for everybody.

- Babies (0 a year)
- Young kids (12-year and a half)
- Older kids (year and a half and up)
- Preschool-age kids (27 months and more established)
- Infant latrine preparing: 0 a year

It sounds abnormal to a ton of Westerners. For guardians in nations like India, China, and East Africa, the commonplace potty-preparing period is youth.

When the infant is all set, the dad holds him over a sink, a bowl, a restroom, or an open field. As the infant exhausts, the dad makes a trademark sound or motion.

Guardians frequently forestall a portion of the issues related to the instructing of more established kids. Children are not used to wearing diapers, so they don't have many such examples of breaking. What's more, at its youthful latrine preparing age, the smell of a kid's pee and excrement is less offensive to the vast majority.

When Exactly Does The Training Start?

Generally, potty preparing starts for the initial three months after birth. Be that as it may, a few advocates propose a to some degree later potty preparing time of between 3-6 months when infants pee less frequently and can sit alone. When a youngster can sit upstanding and stable, you can prepare him in a seat to go to the restroom.

It is additionally conceivable to begin later, somewhere in the range of 6 and a year.

When infants find versatility, they're less patient when they're despite everything sitting in a pot. What's more, one author recommends that more seasoned youngsters, as more established kids, have gotten familiar with wearing diapers and disregarding their body signals.

Picking the correct age to go to the washroom for more seasoned infants and little children (12-year and a half)

During the 1920s and 1930s, European and American guardians regularly started preparing somewhere in the range of 12 and year and a half. In any case, contingent upon your kid's character and advancement plan, it could be a tricky potty preparing age.

For one, more seasoned infants and little youngsters may make some hard memories getting out from under the diaper propensity.

Yet, its preparation age has its focal points. Youngsters younger than a year and a half are regularly anxious to satisfy grown-ups. A quality more established youngsters may need (think about the "awful two").

In case you're intrigued, you can attempt the child's potty technique. On the off chance that your kid comes up short, return, and try again later. What's more, keep the targets sensible. The potty preparing period is tied in with remaining dry with near parental management.

If you choose to hold up until your preparation age to go to the restroom later, you can, at present, exploit its second. The 12-18-month span is the ideal opportunity to begin considering setting off to the bathroom.

Proposed signs incorporate formative achievements, such as strolling, the capacity to follow verbal requests, and the capacity to remain dry for two hours one after another. They likewise include new perspectives, for example, "your child says he needs to get things done for himself" and "your child says he needs to wear grown-up clothing."

You are trusting that your kid is prepared sounds sensible. Who's going to make a youngster not readied? The issue lies in the way you characterize your preparation.

Does your youngster need to stroll around to utilize the restroom? Do you need your youngster to communicate enthusiasm for clothing? The appropriate response relies upon your objective.

On the off chance that you likely get your youngster to go to the restroom and sit alone on the pot, at that point clearly, you should hold up until he can walk. If you're keen on the more unassuming objectives of newborn child and baby preparing, you don't have to hang tight for indications of cutting edge "preparation." But regardless of whether your aim is to absolute autonomy from the restroom, you ought to step by step accomplish it.

The more significant part of the kids demonstrated no enthusiasm for utilizing the washroom until the following two years. "Remaining dry for over 2 hours" took over 26 months for half of the kids, and most youngsters couldn't expel their clothing until they were more than 29 months.

All the more critically, latent holding up doesn't enable your kid to plan. If you survey the official agendas, you see that many, if not most, signs might be energized or appeared.

<u>Arrangement Signs</u>

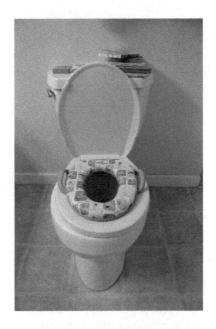

More than once, numerous guardians recognize that they don't have the foggiest idea of how to identify new child availability indications. Here is a portion of the typical signs that your youngster is prepared for potty preparing:

Appears To Be Keen On The Potty Or Latrine

- You are getting keen on observing others go to the washroom (It might be awkward or awkward from the outset, yet it is a magnificent method to introduce things)

- It may incorporate watching him, posing inquiries about the lavatory, or sitting in the restroom.

- Show enthusiasm for the washroom when another person is utilizing it.

Worldwide Prepping Abilities, In Any Event, When You're Not Keen On The Washroom Yet

- Able to walk and sit alone for brief periods

- You can unwind and get up from a seat to go to the restroom

- You can balance out with your feet so you can push when you empty.

He Impersonates His Folks At Home.

- Begins to show a craving to please guardians

You Can Take Care Of Things Back.

- Shows comprehension of things that have their place in the home.

- You are commonly turning out to be freer with regards to finishing undertakings

- Desire to be self-governing

You Have Evaporated Diapers For Two Hours.

- It shows you can store pee in your bladder (which discharges naturally in littler infants or babies)
- Must have the option to rests without a jug or cup

You Have Healthy, Smooth, And Framed Solid Discharges.

- Even if the intestinal cycle isn't yet normal

Ready To Convey Your Desires

- Not even through words, yet through body developments, looks, outward appearances, hand motions.
- Can comprehend and adhere to essential directions, for example, "Give father the ball."
- Understand the words utilized for disposal.
- Tells you (or gives clear indications) when you crap or pee in your diaper or are going to.

It can begin with physical uneasiness, which transforms into curving and turning, at that point, little sounds and words, correspondence, and pre-language.

Awkward With Wet Or Filthy Diapers

pter 1: Complains about moist or messy diapers, or performs activities, for example, expelling diapers and peeing on the floor

pter 2: Report that your diaper is wet or sloppy. A kid should be soggy and feel sodden and awkward to understand that he ought to go to the washroom and reveal to him when to go.

pter 3: You can even request to transform it when the diaper is soiled or attempt to get the crap out of your diaper

pter 4: Begins to know that a diaper is going to get wet, seeing it before peeing

pter 5: Sometimes, in any event, requesting clothing or declining to put on a diaper

pter 6: You can likewise pull your jeans down and back on with practically no assistance.

Not these signs ought to be available when your youngster is prepared. Most youngsters even show a couple of these signs. An overall pattern tells you that.

Introductory Stage

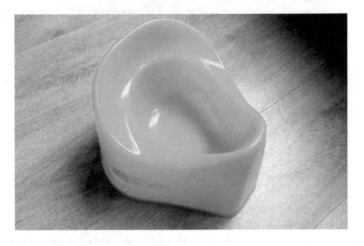

First of all, it is essential to note that all children autonomously wish to use the potty eventually. Whether It happens with 18 months or four years depends on your child's character and the guidance you have given them on how to use the potty. After all, no child wants to go to kindergarten in diapers. However, they may still be accident-prone unless you use its window of the developmental urge to teach them to transition into the toilet use.

The party isn't always that the hands-on as you might think. It isn't about fourth thinking of going to the toilet or announcing that they now are using" new equipment." Instead, you should ease your child into the idea and should reduce your child into the concept so that the change may feel instinctive.

It requires both therapy and a consistent push. You might feel that your child is not internalizing your potty directing probes.

How To Get Your Child To Show Interest

Developing an interest in the potty or the toilet be the first step in your child's transition. They need to conceptualize the bathroom as a necessary component of every person's life. They have to know that they cannot go around toilet use; however, challenging and complicated it may initially look. They should also gauge, from early on, that there are several advantages to using the potty.

Typically, you want to introduce the idea vocally at first. The sound of the parents' voices is, to a child, the first source of probing or advice they may receive in their developmental journey.

Therefore, you shouldn't underestimate its power. Your child is likely to want to please you by relating to any concept you are to mention. You find that your child attributes much interest to the things you might do at work, self-care, or even your home chores. By introducing the topic of potty training, you familiarize them with sharing code of behavior with members of their family and, later on, community.

You want to mention potty training around your child's first birthday occasionally. It is the stage at which they are fully capable of understanding most of your guidance and suggestions; however, they do not remember its settings. Therefore, they are likely to have forgotten their earlier childhood by the ages of two and above. The things you mention around the first birthday likely to eventually strike the child as a mere "instinct."

It is precisely what you should want. It allows your child to perceive specific codes of behavior as innate. On the other hand, brutish mention of the changes they must make it feels like pressure and overwhelming discipline. The latter can make a child lose trust in their parent or guardian to sense that they are being pushed towards performing actions they may not want to. It can be incredibly difficult to undo any later developmental stages, such as pre-pubescence and adolescence.

To make positive mentions of the potty, link it to concepts your child may be familiar with and enjoy. For example, you may want to make the potty or "has to go peepee." You also want to humanize the concept by making mentions such as "mummy has to go use the grown-up potty." It can eventually help them feel safe in the use of the "baby potty."

You should also consider the use of literature searches children's books and audio or video stories mentioning potty use. The less foreign a concept seems to your child, the more open they be in engaging with it. The children's books are the perfect opportunity for you to bond with your little one while introducing the topic they need to master later.

Your attitude around the subject is likely to affect how much interest your child displays. Excitement and joy when discussing the party and communicating the sense of relief that results from going to the toilet, are likely to intrigue your child. It is the curiosity you need to seize to make the transition.

Take It Step By Step

By the time your toddler is ready to potty train, he or she is likely to be able to spend prolonged hours without waiting for their nappy. It is a positive development. It means that your child is in a more magnificent come round of their body as a whole. You need to communicate it to your bundle. It is the first step in establishing toilet training as a transition to autonomy and independence. If your baby is capable of going through an entire nap and waking up dry, spending a couple of hours without wetting their nappy, they are probably ready to advance. It is the time at which you need to congratulate your child on their growth. We feel compelled by your encouragement to impress you further.

Positive progress can be rewarded with anything, from toys to extra affection. After a couple of months of pointing out positive momentum, your child may be more open to the possibility of a transition.

Your next step is to choose the potty and the placement of the potty best suited to your child's needs. It isn't in frequency for children to be anxious about the sound of flushing, the proximity of water, and the size of the opening of a traditional toilet. Such as children often be more comfortable with conventional potties, which can be placed anywhere from the bathroom to your child's room, or even the playroom. Your child also requires a stepping stool in most cases, whether using a traditional potty or a potty seat on top of a conventional toilet. According to Scott J Golf Stein, MD, at the Feinberg School of Medicine at Northwestern, it is impossible to poop without pressing your feet on the floor. Its pressure is required to summon a bowel movement. Without it, children are not able to push comfortably.

Once your child is familiarized with the potty, you may want to introduce a potty seat to place on your traditional toilet in your bathroom. It potty seats make your child more comfortable with the use of the more imposing toilet.

Your next step involves scheduling. Experts claim that it can be psychologically traumatic for a child to be potty trained to do during a stressful period of their life. If your family is undergoing any significant change, it is not the right timing for potty training. If you or partner are facing any personal or work issues that may spill over onto your home life, you may want to delay potty training. Parents always feel that they may squeeze it stage in any busy rocky period of their lives because of the technical possibility of training their child to use the potty within under a week. However, evidence has shown quite the contrary. For the potty training to stick, your child needs a serene period to experiment with his or her newly learned skills.

When starting the actual potty training, you need your child to have already moved out of the crib and into a big kid bed. Because you are teaching your child autonomy from the beginning of the training, you need them to access the potty at any time of the day or night. It means that they need to be able to reach it on their own, even in times of strain or exhaustion, such as in the middle of the night. If you feel like your child is not ready for a grown-up bed, you may want to keep the diapers on for a little longer.

Your next stage is to use the demonstration stage partly. In its stage, you need to implement the potty training methods you have established to be best suited. We advise the schedule method. Its approach is relatively simple; it requires only a rigorous pattern to work effectively.

You need to establish times, preferably every two hours, where your child be required to sit on the potty for a few minutes (around 20). Its time, they try their hardest to "go.". The key to its functioning effectively is to ensure the child is not bored during its time. Prepare books, games, and videos to enjoy with your child during its time as he or she waits for the urge to use the potty. Even if they do not manage to use it, you should advise to wash their hands, flush the toilet, and, most importantly, congratulate them for their effort.

Its ritual may feel tedious and tiresome to the child. They may even want to revert to diapers. You are tempted to give It request a definite no. However, research has found that it may be best to allow your child to have a temporary break from the potty rather than eradicate it.

Such a brutal, absolute change may encourage your child to withhold bowel movements to avoid the potty experience. It can lead to constipation and a very digestive excretion problem. Therefore, you want to work on a compromise with your child by wearing the diaper in the morning or straight after naps. You have to remain firm with the timings you have chosen with your child. Your child is likely to attempt to negotiate to stretch the periods of nappy wearing longer. However, by implementing a reward system, you ensure they are comfortable returning to the potty.

Your reward system should congratulate any potty use. Good handwashing, proper flushing, and pants-pulling all deserve rewards. Think of fun, simple methods such as stars and stickers, which can amount to a real prize: a cake baking session, a new toy, sometimes at the pool, et.al.

Many children still wet the bed thoroughly into the ages of 5 or 6. Nightly accidents are common up until mid-primary school. However, disciplining your child for having a slip is likely to traumatize them.

Let's Get Started

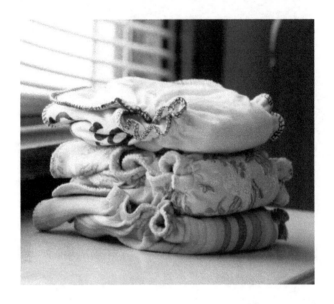

We are potty training, so it is pretty clear that we are going to have to get rid of those diapers. Day one was spent naked, so we didn't need an alternative, but day two could be spent on clothing. That means you may want to introduce underwear. Some parents are okay with putting their child in training pants during potty training and for a while after, and others swear by putting them straight into underwear; what you choose much depends on you and your child.

Even still, putting your kid in underwear isn't as easy as it may sound. And it isn't just hard on your child. It's hard on you as well. You know you are putting them in something that has virtually no protection against accidents. That means your couch, your car seat, and the carpet at your mother-in-law's are all at risk of being peed on.

Your child has developed the muscle memory to their diaper. They have been in that diaper since the day they were born. They are used to having it at their disposal, and they feel safe with it on. When it comes to potty training, they have spent two to three years in peeing and pooping in their diapers. But, guess what also feels like a snug-feeling diaper.

That's why parents who end up transitioning too quickly experience a whole lot of accidents. The kid doesn't understand that underwear is different than their diapers. For a child, their underwear's snug feeling is similar enough to wear a diaper that it is pretty much an automatic response.

With all that said, there are clues to look for in your child and a transition that you can try to make their transition into underwear easier.

How Well Are They Pottying?

Your child may be using the potty reasonably well, but is it mostly at your request? Do they tell you to go, or are you still taking them every few minutes or hours? It is best to wait until they have started to let you know when they need to go because that means they have learned how to recognize the urges in their own body. You may experience something that not many parents experience. Some children refuse to wear diapers anymore, for whatever reason, and that would be your biggest clue that they are ready for the transition into underwear.

Pull-Ups, Training Pants, Or Underwear

Most people have some pretty strong opinions about what toddlers need to wear when they are potty trained. Decide what's the best for your child. Whether or not you should use pull-ups or other disposable training pants depend on your child's age, personality, and situation and how well you can manage accidents. You likely won't know which be the best option until you get into the thick of it. Things to think about:

Training Pants

While your child may use the potty and is happy to oblige you when you ask them to, they may still be too young to have complete control over their bladder functions. It could cause them to get upset when they accidentally wet themselves. Pull-ups or washable training pants could be a good idea to start with.

They are good to use because:

Chapter 7: They can help them get through the night

Chapter 8: They prevent messes when accidents happen

Chapter 9: They can boost motivation in some

Chapter 10: They provide your kid with a "big kid" feel

Chapter 11: They are a better option for toddlers who don't have full bladder control

They aren't a good option because:

Though, training pants are a definite step up from them wearing diapers, and most toddlers like the sound of being a "big" kid. While disposable training pants can end up being a crutch for some, since they are a lot like diapers, if your child is already motivated to be potty trained, they likely won't be. They are a safety tool that can keep your child from getting upset with themselves for making a mess.

They also prevent any big messes that you may have to clean up around the house during the training process and until your child gets the hand of pottying.

That said, there are washable training pants, as mentioned earlier. They help protect from messes and have all the benefits of pull-ups, but they also allow your child to wear underwear. They are waterproof underwear that goes over the top of their regular underwear. If they have an accident, all you have to do is wash them, which can be done in the washer or by hand. They dry quickly so that you can reuse them more often.

Underwear

Since most children aren't ready to start training until after two years of age, they may be prepared to jump right into underwear. These older children also tend to be hard to get motivated for potty training because they have a more robust independence streak, and praise and reward charts might not work well. That also means that pull-ups are likely the wrong decision, at least when it comes to daytime training.

While some children feel the wetness and realize that they have started to pee and run straight for the bathroom, others are perfectly okay with sitting in soiled or soaked training pants for as long as they have to so that they can continue to play with their toys.

It is where cloth training pants that absorb part of the wetness but then transition into regular underwear could be a better option. When they have an accident in thing cotton underwear, the only choice is to stop playing and get cleaned up. It alone is typically enough to motivate the otherwise engaged child to notice all of the signs that they need to get to the bathroom.

Regular Underwear May Be The Best Choice For Your Child If:

Chapter 15: Your toddler seems to need a push. If you are positive that they are developmentally ready to be toilet trained, but they aren't interested in giving up the convenience of using their diaper, introducing them to underwear that is exciting to them, think superheroes, and requires them to use the toilet if they want to keep them can be the best motivator.

Chapter 16: Having to deal with messes isn't a big deal to you. Accidents often upset a sensitive child, so you may want to think about choosing something with a little more absorbency if accidents easily defeat your child. Clean up any accidents that likely happen when you first start training.

Chapter 17: Your toddler is telling you that they need to use the bathroom or go on their own, and they don't require constant prompting and reminding.

One last thing you should think about when choosing between pull-ups and underwear is cost. Pull-ups and other such brands end up costing more than regular diapers, so they are a lot more expensive than a couple of packs of cotton underwear.

After dealing with potty training for one day, you have likely learned what type of potty trainer they are going to be like. To help you transition into underwear, we look at the five main types of trainers and how to handle them.

The Puppy

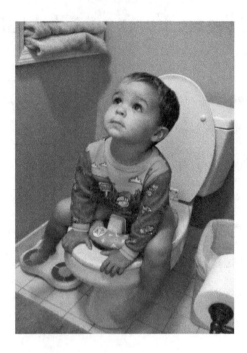

These trainers are the ones that feel confident, and they often make it on their own to the potty before they poop or pee. They are the ones that are the readiest for underwear and make the transition more positively if they continue to feel that Mom and Dad are respecting their potty training timetable.

The time that you spend with them picking out their underwear is a bonding time. The emotional connection you can form with them is the point to be helpful at later stages in their life. Let them pick out where they keep their new underwear. You can say something like, "Where would you like to keep your special new underwear? I keep mine in a drawer. Let's find a place for you."

When they put them on, you can say something like, "Wow! You have big kid underpants on! Can you show me how they work?"

When it comes time for them to use the potty with their underwear, you can try saying things like:

"New underwear is for kids who know a lot about the potty already. Keep doing a great job, and remember to try and notice what your body is letting you know so that you can make sure you make it to the toilet in time to keep them dry."

"Anytime you think that your body may be telling you that you need to go, even if it is just a little bit, you should go try to use the potty. Even if nothing happens, it is always a good idea to try."

When the time comes that they do have an accident in their new underwear, the calmer and more relaxed you can be responding to It, the better. It helps to keep your little one calm as well.

The Turtle

These kids are the ones who don't do too well when being introduced to a new routine. If they get moved into something new too quickly can create a setback. You want to wait until they show more confidence before you try to get them into underwear. They likely take better to wearing pull-ups since they are similar to diapers.

The Owl

It is a child who likes to see their options. They likely are doing pretty good at keeping their diaper or pull-ups dry and go the bathroom with confidence. You can then introduce them to underwear. Explain to them what the differences are between them. Show them side by side. Let them know that they are worn the same way and pull them up and down. They pick up reasonably quickly and likely show an interest in taking the next steps in potty training.

The Squirrel

These kiddos don't have time to waste on focusing on what you are saying. Once they have shown that they can focus long enough to use the potty when they need to, you can introduce them to big kid underwear. They either want to help you shop, or they won't be able to focus on helping you buy. Either way, make sure you get them plenty of styles, colors, and designs to keep them interested.

The Bear Cub

The child is very independent and probably won't be as excited for underwear as the others. It is because they perhaps prefer the idea of filling up their diaper or pull-ups is better than interrupting their playtime to go to the bathroom. Don't worry, though; they become interested in underwear.

After Potty

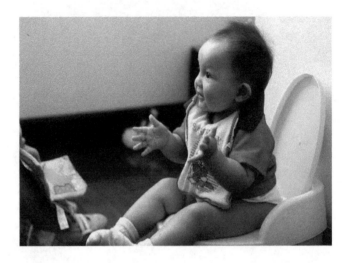

Step 1: Always Be Celebrating

You've passed the first three days of potty training. Congratulations! Keep praising and rewarding your child. You may be tired of pretending to be as excited about pee as you would be about winning the lottery, but trust me, your child isn't tired of it.

Because you still want your child to feel motivated to use the bathroom, it's best to wean her gradually from the attention and rewards instead of cutting her off entirely. Usually, the sticker chart is the first reward to go because she starts to forget about it. Keep the sticker chart up for the initial three days, and when your child starts forgetting about it, stop reminding her.

Since the food treat is usually the key motivating factor to potty training, continue to give it to your child for at least two weeks—and even longer for pooping on the potty. If, after two weeks, you feel your child has the hang of peeing on the potty, stop giving her a treat if she forgets to ask for it. Your child may remember a couple of times, which is okay, but after two days, you should say, "I'm so proud of you for being such a big kid. You get two treats for pooping on the potty, and that's how you can get treats now. Please tell me when you have to go potty."

Step 2: Family Members And Other Caregivers

One way to confuse your child and make the potty-training process take even longer is by not having everyone who takes care of your child on the same page. If you have gotten it far in the book, you most likely choose its method to use when potty training your child. Any person who is with your child in the bathroom should become knowledgeable about its plan. I have seen more than one argument between parents when they read the project and the other parent has not. Don't let that be you.

Partner Up

Communicate with your partner. If you have been the one potty training your child at home, you know your child's cues and have a whole method down with her in the bathroom. Your partner may not have had as many opportunities to be involved with the process. Be patient. If your partner keeps an eye on the child while you shower or run errands, explain the specific things to look for when your child might have to go to the bathroom, and some things to avoid, such as letting her watch TV or play on the iPad.

At School

Your child's teacher is in to help as much as possible and be a significant part of your support system, but unless the school has a potty-training program, it is not the teacher's job to potty train your child. It takes time for your child to get used to going to the bathroom in a different place, with another person, and with other procedures, so let your child's teacher know what kinds of things to do or say to help your child keep her underwear dry.

Let your child go to the bathroom she uses at school as soon as you drop her off. Doing it gives her the chance to go to the bathroom with you, the person she's most comfortable with, which makes her feel more comfortable using the school's bathroom. Not only that but knowing she has emptied her bladder at the beginning of the school day means she should be able to stay dry for a couple of hours, which helps the teacher know when to start giving your child extra bathroom reminders.

Everywhere Else

It's always a good habit to bring a newly potty-trained kid to the bathroom immediately upon arriving at any new location. Nothing is worse than getting halfway through with grocery shopping, only to have your child tell you she needs to go to the bathroom.

Step 3: Naptime And Nighttime

The keys to staying dry at night are an empty bladder and no fluids two hours before bedtime!

The only time I use pull-ups during potty training is while a child is sleeping, and I usually recommend using nighttime pull-ups, which are different than regular pull-ups. I know, telling you it's okay to use pull-ups seems contradictory to what I said earlier. Still, I find it extremely unfair to expect a two- to three-year-old to stay completely dry during training, especially if she cannot get up using the bathroom herself in the night.

So, here are my tricks for continued success:

1. Call these pull-ups "sleeping underwear."

   That way, your child still believes they are related to underwear.
2. The sleeping underwear goes on right before getting into bed.

   Avoid wearing diapers, which is the opposite of what we are trying to accomplish here.

3. The sleeping underwear comes off immediately upon waking.

> Well, within a minute or so. You don't want to give your child enough time to wake up and pee in it.

4. 4. Your child's regular underwear must go on top of the sleeping underwear—every time.

When your child looks down, she should see underwear. It is a mind trick. Your child has been trained to use the bathroom while in her underwear, and for the most part, she continues to do so even while sleeping. Of course, accidents happen, and bladders need time to train.

If your child still takes a nap (wow, you are so lucky!), It is the testing ground to see how well she can control her bladder while sleeping. Kids can keep themselves dry for a nap way before they can stay dry all night—naps are much shorter.

an empty bladder

Nighttime fluids are always a touchy subject with parents; many who come to me still give their kids sippy cups filled with milk before bed to keep their belly full overnight. They are often afraid that cutting back on the dairy may disrupt the child's sleeping patterns, but there are other ways to fill a kid's belly before bedtime.

Be patient with your child during its overnight process. Each child develops differently, so make sure your child knows there is no shame in having an overnight accident.

Step 4: Accidents

No one wants their child to backslide with potty training less than I do. It makes me look bad. However, some extenuating circumstances may cause some potty-training troubles, such as:

Never be angry or upset at your child if accidents happen. There is always a reason a child has an accident—whether you weren't paying attention to the warning signs, she didn't want to stop playing with her toys, or there was a new teacher at school she didn't feel comfortable enough with to tell when she needed to go to the bathroom. If you can pinpoint the reason behind your child's accidents, you can find other ways to support her and get her back on track.

One trick to be aware of is your child using bathroom-related things to manipulate you—for example, coming out of the bedroom soon after being put to bed because she "has to go potty." One hundred percent of the time, parents fall for this. (You had her go pee immediately before she got into bed, right?) If you know she peed five minutes ago, then you will know she is playing you. If you realize you forgot to have her sit on the potty before going to bed, then her potty plea may be legit. Accompany her to the bathroom, either way, so you know if she did need to go. If nothing comes out, tell her you to know she didn't have to go, and next time will be different.

Step 5: Keep Teaching

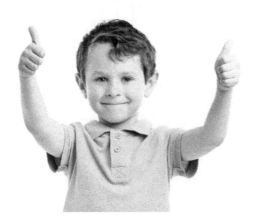

Yay, you've gotten almost to the end of its potty-training plan, and hopefully, it was successful! After three days of potty training, you should have laid a great foundation. Follow through and give positive reinforcement. With each passing day, it should become more comfortable and more accessible, and once your child is four years old, she should require minimal assistance in the bathroom.

We never stop teaching our children, so other things you can teach them to include:

pter 27: »How to step up to the toilet themselves

pter 28: »How to wipe themselves

pter 29: »The proper way to wash their hands

pter 30: »How to pull up their underwear and pants

You're about to be amazed at the transformation your child achieves. Parents tell me how big their child looks now that she is potty trained, and your child is about to show you how big of a kid she is now.

What to Do

Tips And Techniques For Potty Training

Girls need to sit down to pee or poop on the potty. Boys need to sit for poop, but when they pee, most stand up. Because of its slight biological disparity, it may be a more straightforward job to motivate and support your boy child to use the potty! Think about:

Chapter 31: Shooting or aiming for something takes effect. When a little boy begins to urinate in a standing position, get ready to wipe around the toilet and on the seat-and often!

Chapter 32: Teach the boy how to aim down his penis to prevent flooding the space, either seated or standing up.

Chapter 33: Show the boy how to target accurately by making him drop items suspended in the pool. It may be a corner of an envelope or a strip of toilet paper, but we find floating Cheerios or Froot Loops is even more enjoyable and aims for the opening

Chapter 34: Remove the water from the toilet bowl and mark a red target on the porcelain backward using a fingernail polish or red grease marker. Let him hit the bulls-eye.

Chapter 35: The urination of bowel water into the "blue" toilet turns it green. (It fits for children, also, although it is more challenging to see.) You may even use coloring food in its method. Red or blue food coloring transforms orange or green as the liquid sprays it. It can be too much fun having your kid do magic tricks on his body fluids!

Chapter 36: Let a boy practice his target in the summertime and the safety of a backyard or woodland. • Let the sons and fathers have a "peeing party."

Chapter 37: Let a boy "write in the snow" during winter.

Chapter 38: If a kid tries to rise but has to be a bit bigger, stay behind him and make him balance on your foot.

Chapter 39: Make sure that in those early stages, the toilet seat cannot fall on a young boy. Let your child verify whether the place is tightly up until urinating.

Chapter 40: Start teaching your son that after he is finished, the toilet rim needs to be put down.

Finally, we have some general tips that do not fit into any specific category. If we repeat ourselves, we are sorry, but potty training is a serious affair, so they are happening!

In General

Here are some ideas and thoughts falling into that general category of collection. Here is a wealth of information. See when the toilet seats start tilting. Some positions are inclined to fall rapidly when placed upright. If the seat tilts or has to be manually supported, change it. The chair has to stay up, so it does not fall and strike the penis of a boy when he is standing up urinating. If your kid is fond of unrolling the toilet paper, consider it. Squash the roll until you place a fresh turn on the roller so that the interior of the cardboard roll is no longer reliable. It way, it does not unroll as easily. It often does not get too much paper per pull on the sheet for the little ones that are potty training.

Play potty as a stuffed toy or doll is in school. Use the future underwear your child has on the animal. Since the underwear is through, showing the child how to pull trousers down and up would be more straightforward. Playhouse with your brother, and imagine. You are the mum of an animal. Feed the cat, make it sprint to the potty, pull down trousers, sit down, maybe read a book to it, thank it for trying/performing, scrub, pull up shoes, flush, and wash face. Act it out again. Let your child be mum and take the animal with you, if necessary, to offer corrections through the steps. Listen carefully to the terms that your child uses here. You should also use the same words later, while you are the true Mommy again! Replicate. Devoting time with excessive repetition here can bore you but gives your child excellent instruction. To make it even more fun, introduce some fun songs and dances here! Try to wear a wet doll. It is a tip that is suggested by renowned psychologist Dr. Phil. Dr. Phil tells having an anatomically appropriate doll that wets let you illustrate how to go potty with the kid. You may want to start emptying poopy diapers into the bathroom, instead of only tossing them out. You're teaching your kid that It is where the feces belong and that he or she would be less prone to letting go of that during the bathroom exercise. Recall that a human being is mental, making up is incredibly complicated. It is not fair to expect a kid to have a limited set of feelings only because he or she is low in stature.

Look out for someone to mess with. Through playing on perceptions and assumptions, siblings may set a child off; peers or even teachers can do the wrong thing. Draw a picture of your child in a bathroom. Ask for clarity about something you do not understand. You might get some clues about worries or fears that the child has repressed. Its cycle actively avoids using pull-ups or diapers. Throwing away the diapers can help make more of what you know for practical potty training. Your child sees when you make a big production of it that it is time to let go of that part of their lives. If you use pull-ups, it looks like your kid wears a diaper. You permit them, in a way, to use that pull-up as a diaper and to wet it in. They learn that way. Do not seesaw from diapers and pull-ups and pants for weeks and months. To infants, it is confusing, and it just destroys their feelings of self-esteem. (It is okay to use pull-ups for a few weeks at night while your baby works on their physical control, but do not use them during the day.) If your baby has been sitting on the pot for 5 minutes without any results, give it up. Try on another time again. Having them sit there that long is plenty of time to see if they can expel their waste or not. Keeping the child on the pot for more prolonged only causes frustration and boredom!

Another potty training idea is to make sure your child has clothing that is quick for your child to put off. Although it may be easy for a mom to put those cute shorts on her child, it may be too hard for your kid to pull down. Try to look at things as your baby would: It is the best tip you can find on potty training. When you select cotton while purchasing training pants, let your child choose his / her favorite ones (Rugrats, Superman, Barbie, et al.). Cotton training pants can help your Child sense the heat and learn more rapidly. The downside is they are just messier! Disposable training pants are easy to clean and go, but if your child does not feel the discomfort of wetness, it may take longer to train. If you buy cotton, you should buy more than one pack of three.

You go through these quickly and want to have plenty in your diaper bag and dresser. Toilet training can get messy, so prepare yourself and expect many mistakes to be made. Your child is learning a challenging skill. Clean up any accidents without feeling angry or indignant. Do not report harshly. Let your child help you throw the slides out of the trashcan. Shop now for new underwear together! Dress your child in easy-to-take and-out clothes. Do not threaten your baby by holding him/her in soiled or damp diapers.

Spring and summer are excellent toilet train occasions. Without his / her diaper, let your child watch them notice their body functions when they can see just what came from when they can get a more definite sense of what they are doing! We cannot emphasize its aspect deeply enough: do not let your kid stay against his or her on the toilet. Make sure that the wardrobe for your child is adaptable to the potty training.

To put it another way, maintain a strategic distance from overalls and shirts that snap into the groin. Straightforward garments are fundamental at their stage, and kids should have the option to uncover themselves when they are potty preparing. Be sure that all professions of your kid embrace a similar calendar that you have set up. Let them see what you are doing and how you tackle any difficulties you may discover. When your youngster is with them, request that they utilize those equivalent strategies so your kid won't be bewildered. Try not to believe that latrine preparation is unthinkable because your kid is in childcare. Studies have demonstrated that you can prevail in potty preparing together as long as you are in consistent contact with your childcare supplier regarding your systems! On the off chance that you stay up with the latest on what you are doing to enable your kid to turn into a latrine prepared, they can do similar strategies significantly more agreeable while they are with you and fortify all that you have concentrated on! Try not to get everyone up to speed with the negative implications that numerous grown-ups have about the human body. Latrine preparation is a piece of an in-depth rooted learning process about the association and how it capacities. The mentalities of adults towards private parts and the normal latrine preparing process affect the kid's creating emotions about her or his body and assuming liability for real needs. Ensure a parent or believed grown-up has watched the kid utilizing the restroom. Answer inquiries in a more loosened up way.

Latrine preparation performed serenely and decidedly is necessary for the valuation of human sexuality all through life. Little youngsters feel the delight of peeing or having a stable discharge. They may wish to play with their pee or with their excretion. They may likewise need to investigate the privates of their own or other youngsters when utilizing the restroom. It is an exploratory conduct, which is typical. The educating of right names for body parts and body capacities is a decent time. The point is to instruct kids that all body parts are correct and that body capacities are regular. The absolute best counsel originates from individuals who were there, and they did that.

What Are The Psychological Effects Potty Training?

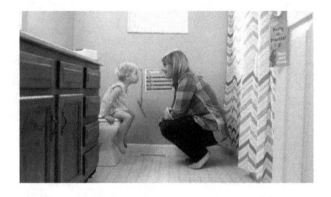

Potty training is a crucial developmental stage in all children's lives. It is a time of transition for most kids into their first sense of autonomy. However, it's also a period of vulnerability for the toddler, who is thrust into a new routine and challenging expectations seemingly overnight. Therefore, simple parental slips can have drastic effects on children.

Calm and patience can typically prevent your child from developing psychological trauma during potty-training. You have to find ways to remain serene and hopeful, even in the most chaotic stages. It is your responsibility, as a parent, to protect your child from the likely sentiment of helplessness he or she is expected to develop. It would help if you remembered that their desire to excrete was hardly put under a microscope; instead, their needs were tended and then catered to.

As your child attempts to find their way into the "big-kid" kingdom, they look to you for reassurance and protection. An inability to empathize and a short temper is going to shock and frighten them. We examine the "tricky" situations which may arise from potty training. We also discuss simple, healthy ways of dealing with them.

Remember that potty-training is less about regiment and routine than your bond with your child and your level of confidence in yourself. Like many other parents, however, you have to learn how to manage your emotions to protect your child from possible psychological trauma.

Potty-Training And Erikson's Psychosocial Theory Of Development

Erik Erickson was a praised psychologist who believed each child went through 8 major stages of development. These stages apply incredibly well to the potty-training experience.

The trust versus mistrust stage involves confusion about whether or not to welcome change. Crucial transitions are often judged by children based on who proposes them. However, even their mommy or daddy may not immediately earn their trust. They have to gradually be reassured that their parents have their best intentions at heart.

Similarly, your child may float between autonomy and shame at early potty-training stages. They carve the sentiment of independence stemming from being able to use the potty or toilet by themselves but also experience shame when unable to manage said autonomy.

Successful Vs. Unsuccessful Potty Training

It is incredibly rare for potty training to be unsuccessful in a healthy child. Most often, a perspective of what defines successful potty training requires a little bit of editing. Most parents believe that successful potty training is completed in a couple of days; however, there is evidence to suggest that the process as a whole may take much longer. It would help if you only changed your outlook on the training experience itself. It isn't because your child is feeling to use the potty that they have not to internalize. There need to do so. They may be more aware, or insurance, with their need to use the blue, but only lack of excellent motor skills. Most parents believe that successful potty training is completed in a couple of days; however, there is evidence to suggest that the process as a whole may take much longer. It would help if you only changed your outlook on the training experience itself. It isn't because your child feels to use the potty that they have not internalized their need to do so. They may be more aware, or insurance, with very need to use blue, but like the excellent motor skills to apply the necessary routine.

Sometimes, our children struggle to understand the necessity of changes at a young age. Not all children mature at the same stages or periods of their lives. It is up to you, as a parent, to accept their timeframe. Ironically, a refusal to delay the potty training process upon your child's request may reject the transition.

Children have a full bladder and bowel control by age four. Research has also shown that girls usually complete success for potty training at the earliest stages than their male peers. It usually takes girls only 3 to 6 months to complete potty training with infrequent occurrences of incidence. However, boys can require anything up to 18 months to be fully potty trained. Regardless of these variations, it is essential to note that successful potty training is not a matter of "if" but "when."

There have been various changes to the perspective of how and when to complete successful potty training. In 1932, the US government proclaimed that parents or begin toilet training as early as three months after the birth of the child. The government believed that It would enable children to be fully potty trained by the age of 6 to 8 months. However, it puts children at a higher risk of certain developmental disorders, such as urological problems or anxiety-wetting. Fortunately, there is no evidence that the time you start potty training may have psychological consequences on your child's well-being.

What has mattered the most to researchers has been finding the window of time most auspicious for potty training with one definite promise: your child eventually gets there. But what happens until they do?

You may feel that your potty training attempts have been unsuccessful if your child is doing any of the following:

And yes, it isn't uncommon for children as young as 24 months to "guilt-trip" their parents with the expertise of a psychology expert. According to many scientists, it is because manipulation has been instilled in most humans from early on as a primary means of survival. If you feel like your child is crying for a reaction, or acting warp said that they might be to sway your emotions, you may not be wrong. At such a young age, children cannot discern the importance of emotional honesty around those who love them. They perceive crying or throwing a tantrum as an appropriate means of getting what they want. It is your responsibility as a parent to remain firm, without flipping into cruelty or apathy. For all his or her red-faced anger, your child perceives his or her fit as a mere occurrence in his or her day. Toilet respond well to humor, even when used to satisfy their own overflowing emotions. If you catch your child attempting to sway you away from a rigorous potty schedule using emotional manipulation, laugh it off. However, for your child and not to feel unloved or alienated, you need to involve him or her in its laughter. Encourage your child to see the positive in even the most stressful moment. They may not get what they want to know, but their adherence may earn them a sticker, which brings them closer to a gift or rewards they enjoy for much longer than they do "suffer" on the potty.

Psychological Trauma From Bad Potty Training

Bad potty-training is similar to child abuse in many ways. In both cases, the child is made to feel guilty, helpless, or worthless. It can have long-term psychological trauma on children. Research has shown that children who suffered poor potty-training may have anxiety issues, depression, and relationship issues even in late adulthood due to suffering throughout that stage.

It psychological trauma is often hard to notice at the early stages. Children may behave as if nothing is troubling them until early adolescence. Later pathologies, however, may indicate an old trauma. If you sense that your child may be struggling to cope with your training methods, you may want to:

1. Use a more patient approach to potty-training
2. Consult a psychiatric professional for your Child

3. Offer your child "time-outs" where they may decide to interrupt the potty-training.

Psychological trauma is the result of pain, shock, and fear. Therefore, the less you provoke these sentiments in your child, the less likely he or she has resulting anxiety or depression.

Child's Sense Of Control

Your child's sense of control may be more much more developed than you think. Your child has learned, from an early age, that most of their "reflex" actions lead to reactions which most often benefit them. It may take your child a while to know that they need to get everything they want; no one should expect everything to be easy. It can be alarming for your child, who may feel they are being thrust into adulthood to withhold parental love, care, or protection from them.

Suddenly, you're a baby who may have until then felt like the king or queen of the house feel helpless and weak. It is not improved by the likelihood of accidents or the difficulties they face at the early stages of potty training. The latter is likely to be an insignificant conflict with their sense of identity. It is often the stage where parents can inadvertently instill a sentiment of fear in their children.

When children are potty training and learn that their primary human responses must be adapted to mummy or daddy's schedule, they can easily panic. To balance out Its sentiment of helplessness, you have to allow your child more control in other areas of his or her life.

For instance, you should leave your children more room to choose their daily outfits, the toys they want, or what they want to watch or read. It would be best if you tried to engage in more activities with your child that involve mutual input, like baking, taking a pottery class, or play-acting a favorite story. During these times, you want to encourage your child to participate. It helps your toddler feel valued and in control of an element of your communal life.

Positively enough, you can expect your child to derive a particular pride from the command of their body they develop during potty training. Its sentiment is to be encouraged, as it is well-deserved. It would help if you always nurtured whatever sensibility of autonomy and power your child appears to develop. It is an exciting progression! It prepares your child for a life of their own in a much grander world, which is theirs for the taking.

Don't Spin Your Wheels – Overcoming Potty Problems

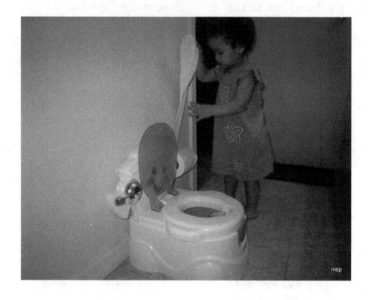

It's been noted that every child is different and work and progress at his or her own pace. Many kids, however, face the same kinds of challenges in potty training. Here are a few quick and simple remedies for some of the most common potty training problems.

My child Won't Stay Seated On The Potty.

First, be sure that any busy activities, toys, and books you're using during the potty time are reserved for that time only.

Second, you can try singing a potty song with your child. It doesn't require you to sit beside your child and help give them a reference for how long they need to relax. Start with just one verse or chorus of a short song and increase each trip to the potty.

If you don't sing, try counting instead. Be sure to take your time getting from one number to the next, keep it lighthearted, and have your child count along with you. In it case, you can either count to a higher number or count slower until your child can sit for 1 to 2 minutes.

Remember, each visit to the potty gets a little longer until your child can sit for up to 5 minutes.

My Child Can Use The Potty But Can't Do It Independently.

Congratulations on having a toilet-trained child! Whether it is a child who can or can't physically manage the potty tasks without help, you need to focus on asking for your child to try first and then ask for help. Praise your child for every step completed independently and add an extra reward, like a mini M n M, for most successful attempts at any task that has not been mastered yet.

My Child Keeps Saying He Has To Go To The Potty But Does Nothing.

It could be that your child has found that he or she gets individual attention from you when going to the potty. If it is the case, be sure you stay out of sight and try not to interact or talk while your child is in the bathroom.

My Child Consistently Uses The Potty But Has Little Accidents Too.

Your child may not be fully emptying his or her bladder when peeing. Try prompting your child to push out a little more after indicating that he or she is done going to the potty. If nothing comes out, finish the routine and return to the bathroom in 10 minutes. Praise your child for going again if he or she goes back, but do not give extra rewards or stickers, as it is just finishing up from the last trip to the bathroom.

Your child has gas. Sometimes when trying to push out gas, a little urine escapes. If you notice a little pee, but not much, it could just be gas. As your child's control gets better, it should decrease.

You may find it helpful to reward your child for staying dry as well. Randomly stop your child and check to be sure that his or her underwear is clean. Reward immediately and give lots of praise for a dry diaper. Do it a few times during the day, and gradually, as your child is more and more successful with staying dry, phase out the check-and-reward system.

My Child Loves To Unroll All The Toilet Paper.

You could remove the paper from your child's reach, but it might remove it from yours when needed. If relocating the roll isn't an option, try putting a piece of painters' tape on the wall.

Teach your child that it's okay to pull down to that line, tear off one piece, and then use it to wipe. Permitting to take some can help keep them from pulling the whole roll off the wall.

My Child Throws A Fit Every Time We Enter The Bathroom.

It could be that your child is afraid of something in the bathroom. Perhaps falling off the seat or the feeling of pooping bothers your little one? If your child is older, you can have a conversation about it, but for younger ones, you may need to reassure that the bathroom is safe and nearby and keep things as light and fun as possible.

It could also be that your child isn't interested in potty training. Sometimes, a child loses interest without warning.

Don't fight it; potty training shouldn't feel like a chore, or your child fights you every time. Take a break and try again when your child starts to show interest too.

My Child Won't Stop Playing To Use The Potty.

It is a prevalent issue for toddlers. Be sure you're informing your child about the progression of events.

Use simple words to indicate that you are only asking for a short break from an activity, like playing with cars.

Say, "first, you go potty, and then play cars!" Repeat it if necessary because, sometimes, it takes your child a minute to process its request.

You can also use a countdown technique to end one activity and start another. You can say, "3, 2, 1… All done, cars! Let's go, potty! Say bye, cars!"

Finally, potty times should come at natural breaks inactivity. It helps alleviate much of the anxiety of leaving something behind because you were already going to move on to the next part of your day.

To stop the child from playing to go, invite them to see the potty reward chart. Act overly excited, if necessary, to get your little one's attention. Then, your child is in the right place to use the potty.

My Child Was Doing Great, But Not Anymore. What Do I Do?

Before getting frustrated, you'll need to think about what's been going on. There could be a few ordinary things going on.

First, has your child been going through a significant growth or developmental spurt?

Sometimes, when kids are working hard growing or learning new things, there can be a natural regression. If you suspect that your child's setback is related to achieving another growth or development process, like switching from a crib to a toddler bed, teething, or a growth spurt, rest assured. It is only temporary. To help combat the setback, you want to ask your child to go at the same transition points you started using initially. Make sure you don't go for more than 2 hours without a potty break. You may find that a week of friendly reminders helps you overcome the hurdle and keep ongoing.

Second, is your child throwing a tantrum rather than getting on the potty? If it hurts to go for one reason or another, it may cause "holding" of bowels or bladder, often causing your child to cry or scream that he or she doesn't want to go. You may want to try increasing morning liquids again and increasing fiber.

The idea here is to soften things up so that it doesn't hurt to go to the potty. If you have noticed your child hasn't had a good bowel movement with regularity, you may want to consult your child's pediatrician.

Finally, don't give up, but don't force the issue either. You can try using a countdown to help your child understand that your trips to the potty be quick (i.e., 10, 9, 8 go, go, go!). You can try using keywords, like "first it, then that" to help transition from one activity to another or try gentle breathing exercises to reduce any stress or anxiety your child is associating with going to the potty. Whatever you do, keep reminding yourself that it is temporary. Try to stay upbeat and positive. It may be possible your little one is just trying to assert some control and independence and happily go back to potting successfully so long as you continue to provide a few extra support.

Dealing With Other Family Members

Trying to get your child potty trained can be thought of as a curse and a blessing. The evil is all the patience and time you devote to its process, while the benefit is no more diapers. Some parents might find themselves thinking:

Chapter 46: If I had someone else who could help motivate my child beside me. I would love to have some help.

Chapter 47: My older child starts feeling neglected because I am spending so much time with the toddler.

Suppose you realize that your older child is beginning to have accidents when you start potty training your younger child. They might begin to refusing to use the bathroom altogether. Most of the time, it is a cry for attention because your attention is spent with your younger child. It is just a type of regression that is relatively easy to fix. You can get them involved with helping train your toddler.

The older children can help. There isn't any need to kneel or make it official. From my experience, older siblings are pleased to help potty train their younger siblings if you can abide by the following tips.

How To Get Older Children Involved

A considerable helper when potty training is use idols that encourage your child to use the potty. Older siblings can give them that role model. Most younger children want to be like their older siblings.

Your older child can help show your toddler what it is like to be a "big kid." They can be very helpful to you. I'm not saying that you should let your older child shoulder the entire responsibility of getting your toddler potty trained. Encourage toddlers to copy their older sibling's actions.

Let them get their "big kid" underwear. Ask them if they want some underwear like "big brother/sister wears?"

Let them help in other activities, too. Tell them that since they are big enough to use the potty, they are big enough to support their older sibling to take care of the family pet. A toddler might want to be like their older sibling.

Tips For Getting Help From Older Children

ter 48: Celebrate family style

Celebrate and make it a family affair if you have small success. Getting your older children involved in potty training could provide your toddlers with a sense of accomplishment. Remember to praise your older children separately for being an excellent role model.

74

Chapter 49: Let older children show toddler how to use the toilet

As long as your older child is okay with it, let them guide your toddler how "big kids" use the bathroom. Your younger child looks up to their siblings and wants to be just like them.

Chapter 50: Spend some alone time with your older child

You have to set aside some time to spend it with your toddler and your older child. They need some time where it is just you and them without anyone else around. Children cherish alone time with one parent because they don't have to fight for your attention. It sounds relatively easy, but it is straightforward to slide it on the back burner. You have to make a point to schedule it into your day. Some parents even have a "date night" with their child or take them out for ice cream or breakfast. Try to enlist the help of a grandparent or spouse who can watch your toddler while you take the other child out for fun. It benefits both of you and not just with the potty training. Most parents find themselves continuing "date night" for as long as their child let them. Children at some time feel it isn't "cool" to be seen out with their parents.

Chapter 51: Your older child isn't the one potty training your toddler

You can't make your older child shoulder the responsibility of potty training their younger sibling. They are there to help you. You are the parent; it is ultimately your responsibility. Your older child feels terrible if you make them think a setback is their fault. Cleaned up accidents.

Even though a bit of sibling rivalry is healthy, it could cause your toddler to regress if they think they can't meet your expectations. Keep in mind that children only potty train when they are physically and emotionally ready. If your child is having a hard time, it might be because it is just too early.

If you notice that your older child isn't enthusiastic about helping you potty train their sibling, don't worry. You could come around or they won't. It's ok if they won't help you. Each child is different. Never punish your child for not being interest in assisting you potty train. Nobody wants to sit in the bathroom all day.

Dealing With A Baby While Potty Training Your Toddler

Potty training a toddler while trying to take care of a baby might seem completely impossible, but it could work in your favor after you have created a routine.

Show them the difference between babies and "big kids." If your toddler is ready to be potty trained, tell your toddler that the baby has to wear a diaper because they aren't a "big kid."

Remember to give your toddler praise for any size achievement. Even though it might make you feel a bit crazy, you can talk to the baby about what their older sibling has accomplished. You can say things like: "When you have grown up like Suzie / Nicky, you be able to use the big potty."

Remember to give your toddler rewards to keep them motivated. It makes it fun for them. It can also help get rid of the feeling like they aren't getting as much attention right now.

No Siblings, No Problem

You can use children of peers, friends, or cousins that have already been potty trained.

My niece, Kimberly, suddenly took a considerable interest in my daughter, Gabriella. Kimberly realized Gabby wasn't wearing diapers, and it meant she wasn't a baby anymore. At family get together, they are close friends. Kimberly loves playing with Gabby more now since she thinks she is a big girl like Gabby.

Potty Training at Two Different Houses

Trying to potty train a child that has to move between homes can be rather tricky. It doesn't matter what kind of relationship you have with your child's other parent, when you potty train, you have to have excellent communication to make sure that you have a successful process. Ways your child gets out of diapers and gets into underwear as quickly as possible.

Chapter 53: Know that you both are ready

Children usually begin to show signs that they are ready to start potty training between 18 and 24 months. It is essential to think about what your child needs while deciding when the best time to start.

Your toddler might have started giving you signs that they are ready to begin potty training without knowing it. Some of these signs might include complaining when their diaper is wet. They get reclusive or fidgety when they have to go or tell you that they need to go potty before they use their diaper.

When you know for sure that your toddler is ready to be potty trained, talk to your co-parent. Ensure that both of you are on the same page about the process so that you can work together.

pter 54: Make sure each house has the right equipment

You want the process to be precisely the same at both houses because It confuses your child and makes potty training harder. Each home includes:

pter 55: Potty training tools like games, books, or shows that talk about the subject.

pter 56: The special underwear you let them pick out above.

pter 57: Extra clothes in case they have an accident.

pter 58: Potty chair, potty seat, and step stool so they can feel like a "big kid."

pter 59: Know what you need for a boy or girl

There are some differences between potty training a girl and a boy. Be an example to your child. Make sure your co-parent knows what to do for each.

For girls: You have to teach them how to wipe the right way so they won't get any infections, which is from front to back. It is vital if they have pooped.

For boys: You need to begin teaching him to sit. It helps him until he can distinguish between bowel and bladder functions. When he can tell the difference, show him how to stand to pee.

Chapter 60: Picture out a routine

When potty training your child, it is essential that they get into a routine no matter where they are. It means you need to have the same expectations at both houses.

Your child has to get used to sitting on the potty even if they don't go each time. Both you and your co-parent have to agree that make the child try to use the potty at the same time every day, especially right before nap time and bedtime.

Whatever the rules and routine you choose, you have to make sure that they stay the same. It includes the points above but how long they need to sit on the potty even if they don't go.

Chapter 61: Use the same words

Potty training can be confusing for your toddler since they might not be able to understand all the new words involved. It can cause a disaster if the terms used in each home are different.

Speak with your co-parent about the words you be using when potty training the child. When talking about body parts while potty training, some people say it is best to teach the child the correct terminology to help instill a sense of body awareness early in life.

You are rewarding your child's achievement, while potty training could be a great way to encourage your child to continue trying. Keep the rewards the same at each house, so your child has the same feelings about potty training.

You can give your child a sticker book that they take from house to house to put stickers each time they successfully use the potty. You can give them one sticker when they pee in the potty and two stickers for when they poop in the potty. You could also offer the child a bigger prize if they use the potty without any accidents for a whole week.

The Most Effective
Method To Keep Your
Potty-Training Methods
Working

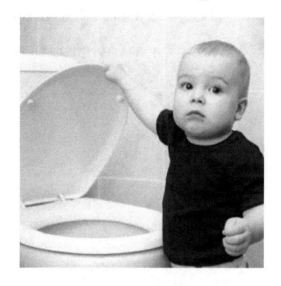

When you potty train a kid, you don't simply stop when you feel like he has learned everything. There are sure things you need to do to ensure that the training becomes part of the child.

Consider it along these lines; assume you were lectured about something new today; would it be implanted in your mind immediately? Likely not, you would unquestionably need to process the information for some time before understanding it.

Along these lines, with regards to potty preparing, you need to ensure that you follow these:

Patience - even when your child says he does not want to go potty. It might just be that he does not want to use the potty yet. Or perhaps, he does not understand what to do, and he is shy. Indeed, it can be disappointing and frustrating, mainly because you know you are merely attempting to do what is best for him.

Despite all of it, you should not spook him by getting angry at him because he refuses to make use of the potty.

Adopt a Laidback strategy - once more, your kid learns better when he feels like potty training is an excellent encounter and that it is not something he ought to be frightened of. At the point when you become so strict or angry, odds are, your kid feels like potty training is frightening or that he is being punished, that is not the sort of thing you need to show.

The primary point is to understand that a kid learns through encouraging feedback rather than being yelled at.

Applaud, laugh - maintain a lively atmosphere for every training session, as you already know, and children are naturally playful. You must acknowledge his effort at all times because it is a good thing that he is trying. The exact moment your kid jumps on the potty seat, feel free to sing his praise. It is an achievement already when the kid thinks that he is being cheered on from the beginning; his confidence in himself increases amazingly. Be the sort of parent who leads and support him at all times.

What to do when you are on the road - whenever you want to hit the road or go on a vacation, you must carry the potty chair along or check if the spot has a toilet that is comfortable for kids, so you can keep practicing. At its stage in your kid's life, you need to be consistent.

Understand that it might be a gradual process - once more, as earlier stated and now being reiterated, training like it requires time. He does not just get it all at once, and it must be at the back of your mind that the training yield results, but not an instant effect.

He may need to relearn some exercises, so it is ideal not to get frustrated, but to show him the procedure again if confused.

Regard your kid's unique learning curve - kids have distinct abilities to absorb information. Some find it easy to learn, while others might take time. If your kid falls in the former, it does not mean that your child is not perfect. He might need time and extra care. The famous Albert Einstein is presumed not to have spoken until he was four years of age, individuals learn at a different speed, and we shouldn't pass judgment.

Never you make the mistake of comparing your kid with others because when you do, it severs and creates a bridge between you. It's time to be patient and realize that your kid eventually learns. Understand the stage he is right now by putting yourself in his shoes.

Be consistent - the law of repetition has made consistency the way to accomplishing nearly everything. Being consistent gives you the room to train your child to do anything, including potty. Follow through on a schedule, and he gets it faster than you expect. When you remember it, things become more straightforward for both of you.

Make a point to go potty fast - presently, when you observe the signs that your kid needs to use the potty or the toilet, regardless if it is outside the schedule, proceed to carry him to their potty spot immediately. Observe if he wants to pee or potty, and if it is out of the program, you don't need to get angry or reprimand him. You ought to feel the need to commend him since he is letting you know or giving you sign that he needs to pee or potty; that alone is enormous progress and a big step towards displacing diapers.

It is ideal for carrying him to his potty spot before sleeping at night, so bedwetting could be maintained strategically, most notably when he is already using underwear. If he needs to pee in the middle of the night, instruct him to wake you up, and please show restraint to get him out.

Pulls-ups or underwear - it relies solely on the kid for it to work, but you must address its issue concerning your kid's character and experience so far with potty training.

For instance, if sure kids are clothed with pull-ups, he may be encouraged to remain and continue playing after the occurrence of accidents. While some other kids might have a feeling of self-pride when they use the potty and when they sense an incoming accident, they hurry to the potty. So, critically analyze your son to know the category he belongs to, but I do not suggest letting him wear pull-ups during the potty training, especially the first couple of weeks. It is based on the fact that it diminishes the kid's drive to make it to the potty.

You can also put the potty training to the test in another environment other than your home. It is because he might just get used to potty at home alone and when in another context, everything changes. So I advise you to brace up for the worst-case scenario while carrying out the trial and error process. I would suggest you use pull-ups for a brief period after your kid has been trained, especially when you are going out. You are introducing underwear to your kid when he is potty trained, and he feels inconvenienced going potty. Get underwear with their favorite character from TV shows or underwear with superheroes on them.

Another thing to consider when it comes to buying or not buying pull-ups is cost. It is an essential factor as pull-ups are costlier than regular diapers, so they are considered temporary.

<u>Signs That A Child Is Already Potty -</u>
<u>Trained</u>

You cannot continue to treat your kid as a potty novice. Some indicators tell us if your kid has fully embraced the potty training. So, how precisely would you realize that your kid is potty-trained already? It is what you must be aware of:

He Knows, And He Let You Know When His Cloth Is Wet

It is an exceptional sign that a kid is as of now potty-trained or is becoming potty trained is the ability to acknowledge that he has wet his underwear. It is an indication of his improved hygienic level, and he realizes there is a need to head off to someplace to use the potty and not merely peeing in his clothing.

He Is Anxious To Get His Prize

Knowing that he is doing something right, the kid wants to prove that he is making progress, and since rewards are used as incentives, he strives to get the prize. It shows you that your son acknowledges that potty training is a good thing. When your kid learns the philosophy of reward and encouraging feedback, he starts to have a competitive spirit. It is something acceptable because it shows that he understands what you're attempting to instruct him. He realizes that he gets rewards when he accomplishes something tremendous and takes a shot.

He goes to the potty seat and attempts to use it, particularly when he has an inclination that he needs to pee or poop. Another enormous sign that he has learned everything and goes for the potty chair by himself. From the beginning, his interest was to please you, but as time goes on, he sees that it is for his good. Furthermore, when he attempts to make the right decision and do the right thing, it implies that he is learning, and you have done well.

He Is Pleased With His New Undies

When you take your baby shopping, and he is excited to get new underwear, that is a good sign. It means he does not see himself as a baby anymore, but as one to take responsibility for his peeing and pooping.

Continue Teaching

Congratulations! Well done! You're well on your way to having yourself a fully potty trained kiddo, which means you're on your way to buying your last pack of diapers! Feel very proud of your child and yourself for how far you've already come! Please remember that everyone's potty training journey is different, so be mindful not to compare yours with anyone else's. The most important thing is that progress is being made, period.

Bittersweet Success

Speaking of progress, here are some examples of how yours might look so far. You see many fewer daytime accidents (if any at all), meaning improved muscle control and greater body awareness. Your child uses the potty when prompted without resistance when in your care, as well as when they're with others. They may even be self-initiating and using public bathrooms occasionally by now. You see, at least a few poop successes, which is no easy feat! And if you've started potty training during sleep periods, your child has some dry naps and nights here and there. I hope. It helps put into perspective the fruits of your labor, all while balancing your already busy schedule!

Consider to be a challenging hurdle in childhood is potty training. At the same time, it's also one of the best ways to instill pride, confidence, and independence in your child. It is a little bittersweet to see your baby growing up, but the pride they exude when mastering its new skill ultimately makes up for the "bitter" part.

Keep in mind that there's going to be a certain level of maintenance and upkeep you'll need to do to keep things moving in the right direction. But the good news is that the basics have been instilled, which means the hard work is done. Soon, you'll be struggling to remember what changing a diaper was like!

Uncommon Issues

Although uncommon, sometimes an event in your child's life can disrupt their potty training progress, even if they were already fully potty trained. Unforeseen circumstances such as injury, illness, trauma (physical or emotional), or anything that results in much stress for your child can cause them to regress.

A potty training regression is when an otherwise potty trained child suddenly starts having multiple, reoccurring accidents. Young children haven't always learned how to process emotion, so it's up to you to help them work through whatever they're feeling. Provide many opportunities to talk and keep the lines of communication open, but don't force them into talking if they don't want to. You always want to validate their feelings by using phrases like "I understand," and "It's okay to feel that way," and "I've felt that way, too." Try to help them look for something positive in the situation. For example, if their emotional stress stems from an injury, say, "I understand you're upset because you can't play soccer. But at least you can eat lots of ice cream until you get better!"

The best thing you can do is to maintain consistency. Go along with your routine as much as possible. Remember, children find comfort in predictability. Do your best to ensure your child is eating healthfully and getting plenty of exercise. Both help them sleep better and balance their moods and emotions. You may need to backtrack in the potty training process a bit as far as to prompt at appropriate times or use rewards for success, but do not go back to diapers. For the most part, regressions clear themselves up within a couple of weeks.

In more severe cases, it may be too much for you alone to help your child cope. If four weeks have gone by, and accidents aren't improving, your child cannot function properly at school or home. You notice any drastic changes in their behavior, or the stress has started resulting in physical discomfort (headaches or stomachaches, for example).

Keep At It

There are many hidden benefits to potty training that are less obvious than ditching the diapers. You also developed new skills for interacting with and caring for your child that you can apply to other aspects of parenting. Continue to utilize what you've learned as your child grows!

The potty training process gets you to think about your child in ways you may not have otherwise. You've probably learned a lot about them: their personality type, how they know, what motivates them, and more. You'll likely find yourself reaching back into your pocket for those tools the next time your child is learning something new—the alphabet, how to write, how to tie their shoes, and lots more. And knowing, really knowing, your child on its level is only going to increase further the bond you share with them.

You've also learned how to help your child adapt to change. With potty training being one of the most significant changes your child has experienced in their little life so far, you probably got a good taste of how they respond to new things. Maybe it was a total breeze, and if it was, that's great! Or perhaps it was a bit of a challenge, or worse. But if that was the case, you learned how to help them come to terms with something new. So now, you can apply those same principles in the future if you experience their resistance toward change.

In addition to getting to know your child, you also learned how to communicate with your child's caregivers and teachers effectively. There may have been much communication among different people to make it a potty training thing a success. And the truth is, it is just the beginning! There are many years of interaction to come with your child's future babysitters, teachers, and coaches. The more involved you are in your child's supervision and education, the better care they receive.

I also hope you've realized how beneficial it is to focus on the successes and, as hard as it may sometimes be, to maintain a positive attitude—not just in parenting, but in all aspects of life. Don't ever hesitate to take a minute to pat yourself on the back. Just as your child deserved praise in their potty training, you deserve it for all of your hard work, too!

Potty Training For Girls

There is no actual training age. However, the average age most parents begin potty training their girls is between the ages of two and three. If your daughter has older siblings, she may learn much earlier than a firstborn.

You should plan your training wisely, specifically opting for the time when no significant changes are happening in your child's environment. If there are substantial changes in the household, wait until she settles down and no longer feels overwhelmed, then begin the training.

If she is at the stage where she says "no" to everything you ask of her, including potty training, remind yourself that she is only in a phase and that once she is through with it, she be receptive to new things. You ought to delay the potty training until the period is over.

Potty Training Equipment

The first step here is to purchase the potty chair or the potty seat and ensure that the child knows that it is hers. It should happen once you notice the signs of readiness, although the training begins weeks, if not months later. Give the child a chance to interact with the potty and learn how it is used. Please encourage your child to personalize the potty by writing her name or placing some sparkly stickers.

Your baby likely feels more at ease training on a potty chair than using the toilet seat right away. Children have a natural fear of falling, and since the toilet is raised high above the ground, the child fears losing to the side, falling on the steps, or falling into the water when seated. It doesn't help that some seats fidget and do not stick firmly to the big chair.

Everything that a child uses must be children-friendly. It should be safe, comfortable, and fun. An excellent potty chair is one that your child can sit on comfortably, move around the house, and sit or rise from it. Besides the comfort and security, a potty chair is advantageous because the child can use it outside of the bathroom, and the parent can empty the contents in the toilet.

You see, bathrooms are dangerous places even for grown-ups, and to have a toddler enter one without supervision when she uses the toilet would be quite risky. Therefore, as you shop, opt for a comfortable light potty chair that she can use unsupervised if you want your child to cultivate some independence so that you do not have to be there or worry whenever she wants to pee.

Since there are some excellent potty-training seats in the market, if your child is not afraid, get her one, and ensure that you make it as easy for her as you can. Ensure that the seat is secure, comfy, attaches firmly, and does not pinch. Get a step stool to make it easier to get to the top of the toilet bowl.

Ensure that you also stock a variety of fun things your daughter can enjoy while using the potty. Stock some picture books, or download a potty-training app for your child to entertain your daughter as she eases herself.

How To Start Potty Training

The best learning avenue for children is via imitation. It is easier for them to do what you do than to follow instructions with your mouth. You may spend much time explaining the potty procedure, and your child won't understand what is happening, but if you demonstrate it, she understands and begin to copy what you do in no time. Therefore, do not close the door when you go in to use the toilet. Leave it open and allow your child to see how it is done.

If daddy does the same and does not lock the bathroom door, your child distinguishes that daddy pees standing up while mummy pees seated. When it happens, please take the opportunity to explain the mechanics behind boys peeing standing up and girls doing it while seated. Tell her that girls and their mommies have to pee sitting.

If she needs a little help, demonstrate how it is done using her favorite stuffed animal or doll. Hopefully, she realizes that using the potty is healthy and quite comfortable.

If your daughter still does not sit on the potty despite your calm efforts, avoid pressuring her because that be the beginning of the power struggle that derail the training process further.

Ways For Her To Use The Potty

The way to get your daughter all excited about potty training is by taking her on a memorable trip to the department store to buy her potty and knickers. Get her some knickers with unique designs and her favorite cartoon characters. Also, ensure that the knickers are comfortable to ensure that your child enjoys wearing them.

Personalize the potty or seat by allowing her to decorate it with some stickers or writing on its sides with some glitter glue. She could use the glue to make interesting patterns. It has her sit on the chair with clothes on for practice. Doing these things should get your child excited about becoming a big girl who can now use grown-up stuff.

The way to build up the excitement is to plan the trip. Get her talking about it every day, and when she does something useful around the house or behaves well, let her know that you reward her when you take her to buy some "big girl stuff" like the potty and the knickers. Tell her that once you begin the training, she starts to be like her elder sisters or like mommy. Keep the hope and excitement alive so that when you finally make the trip, your child be more than excited about purchasing and using the potty-training stuff.

When To Banish Nappies

A child learns and sticks with any skill, so long as presented in her environment consistently. If potty training is made a consistent plan so that the parent, nanny, and the caregiver at the daycare are a coordinated team who uses the same potty-training approach, your child learns the skill much quicker.

The best approach to training is to switch from using diapers to underwear all day, from the very beginning. It way, there be no switching methods in the middle of the training, and your child not be confused. You could also take up the use of pull-up training pants. Still, experts agree that it is the washable cotton training pants that produce the best experience because your daughter is conscious of her wetness immediately when an accident happens. Be prepared that there be several accidents before the child fully masters the use of the potty.

Whenever you are out, carry some clean knickers, pair of tights, and some trousers, even when you are only taking a short trip to the store. Ensure that you leave a more massive stack of the items your daughter could need during the day when leaving her in preschool before going to work. When you leave your child under the care of a nanny or a sitter, ensure that they have quick access to the extra clothes. If you need advice and tips on carrying on the training stress-free, talk to other moms in your playgroup to find out how they solve some of the challenges they encounter. Remember, though, that every child is different and requires a unique approach. Whenever you want to try something new, talk to your child's pediatrician first.

Weeing, Pooping, And Preventing Infection

For girls, even wiping takes a specific strategy. Teach her that she ought to clean starting from the front to the back whenever she uses the potty, especially if she had a poo. It is a healthy practice that keeps bacteria from the bowel spreading into the areas of the vagina and the urethra. If she has difficulty stretching her hand to effectively wipe front to back, opt that she pats herself dry after peeing, and when she poops, she should call for assistance to clean.

A Urinary Tract Infection (UTI) in children, especially girls, is not shared. The disease develops when the child holds in urine for too long, and when bowel bacteria get to the vagina and proceed to the urethra.

UTIs in children are identified through the following signs. The first is that the child begins to complain of pain whenever she pees or some discomfort around the pelvis or tummy region. The second sign is that all of a sudden, the girl begins to wet her pants, even after successful potty training and having achieved reasonable bladder control. The third sign is that the child develops a need to pee more often, and usually, the extreme urge to pee comes suddenly. Rush her to a hospital to treat her if any of these signs occur.

How Can She Recognize The Signs Of Needing A Wee?

Your little girl has to learn how to tell when she needs to go to the potty. You may keep reminding her at the beginning of the training, but with time, she has to be sensitive enough to know when she needs a wee. The way to cultivate its sensitivity is to have your child spend some considerable time during the day without any underwear. It is so that when the pee comes gushing out, the child feels and sees it flow so that whenever the feeling comes, she associates it with wetness and the rush to find the potty.

The potty should always be within your child's reach. Ensure that the distance between the potty and the area from which the child is playing is short to get to it in time. With that said, be ready for the occasional puddles when the child is unable to get to the potty and unable to sit on the potty chair properly, resulting in some liquid drops to the floor.

Have some cleaning agents, such as a carpet cleaner, at hand, or you could cover your carpet with some plastic to keep it from absorbing the fluids.

When To Praise Her During Potty Training

Children love to know that they have their parents' support and approval in all they do. They like to make their parents proud and receive recognition and praise in exchange. Your little girl is like that. She wants to know that she is making you happy and satisfied as she learns how to use the potty. Praise also tells her that she is getting into the "big girl" league, just like mom and the elder sisters. It is a dream come true for her because toddlers like to think of themselves as adults, equal to their mothers and other older people.

CONCLUSION

Thank you for reading all this book!

Potty training can take a long time to accomplish because it is not a one-time event that you teach them to do! In other words, potty training involves many different aspects of a person's life. When a toddler is about to start potty training, they must show some cues, feel ready (you will recognize this as a parent), and comprehend their needs.

All humans are different; therefore, all children will also present other characteristics, feelings, and ways of being. Perhaps you already have a child, and they were potty trained in no time, and it wasn't difficult at all. But your second child is not interested in potty training! We all have different abilities, obstacles, and ways to overcome them.

I hope this book has successfully guided you throughout your potty training journey. It doesn't matter if you are a first-time mom or dad or if you are about to become a parent, and you are looking for information regarding different life stages. This book served you as a guide to know what you should do or say, and what things you should avoid.

This potty training book has also allowed you to see how your child's mind works, so you can completely understand their behavioral, cognitive, emotional, and physical milestones. You will be able to provide comfort and help because you know exactly what is going on with them.

Throughout this book, you also got special tips to implement immediately, from singing funny potty songs, reciting potty poems, or making a special potty dance. As a parent, these are great tips to take into action immediately.

This guide should encourage you to present this new developmental milestone to your child in such an exciting way that they will tell you that they want and need to go potty!

Now you know what to expect and what you can do when you are about to start a potty training journey with a child on the spectrum, or if your toddler has any other special needs requirements.

You have already taken a step towards your improvement.
Best wishes!

CPSIA information can be obtained
at www.ICGtesting.com
Printed in the USA
BVHW091228130521
607269BV00001B/37